YOUR NEXT SHIFT

YOUR NEXT *Shift*

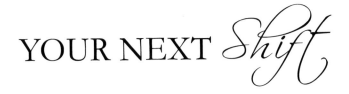

How to Kick Your Nursing Career into High Gear

ELIZABETH SCALA, MSN/MBA, RN

ADVANCED PRAISE

"Finally, a book which talks about the universal laws and how they apply to nurses. Elizabeth Scala eloquently shares her journey of becoming an entrepreneur. She is raw and real and not only discusses her victories but also her challenges and uses these examples as teaching tools to illustrate her points. Using these tools, nurses can get clarity around problems that occurred in the past and how to avoid them in the future.

We can learn from leaders like Elizabeth who have paved the road for other nurses to succeed. Whether you want to advance in your career as a nurse or become an entrepreneur, these tools work because, of course, they are based on universal laws! By embracing the principles in this book, any nurse can create the job they love and be fulfilled in their practice." –Lorie Brown, R.N., M.N., J.D.; Author of 'From Frustrated to Fulfilled: The Empowered Nurses' System'

"This book is like curling up in front of the fire with a friend and cups of hot cocoa. Tired and stressed-out nurses will enjoy Elizabeth's warm advice." - Candy Campbell, DNP, RN, CNL; Author of 'Channeling Florence Nightingale'

"Reading 'Your Next Shift' made me reflect on my own career as a nurse. Elizabeth brings out some strong points on how your mindset matters and your thoughts influence how you feel. She also reminds us there is abundance everywhere, and we should avoid falling into the lack mentality which makes us have fear and worry. A truly inspiring book every nurse should read." –Joyce Fiodembo; Author of 'Reflections and Prayers for Nurses'

"This 'Transformative Textbook' is an amazing practical manuscript with a wealth of inspirational & relevant information. Whether you are a seasoned or an aspiring nurse, the information is so valuable that it will motivate and empower you in your career as well as your unique nursing journey so you will grow to another level. It is packed with valuable, refreshing, insightful, and caring information which is drawn from real life's experience of a great nurse, educator and leader- Elizabeth Scala.

Every nurse from any walk of life who reads this book will be helped and they will advance in their career as well as their leadership." –Eva M. Francis, MSN, RN, CCRN; Author of '*50 Business Ideas for Healthcare Professionals*'

"'*Your Next Shift*' is a powerful resource for nurses who are trying to figure out "what's next?" Ms. Scala provides helpful insights, stories and questions to help her healthcare colleagues dive deeper into what really matters at work and what you can do about it." -Vicki Hess, RN, MS, Certified Speaking Professional; Author of '*SHIFT to Professional Paradise*'

"The author, Elizabeth Scala, NAILS it!!! The void in the market for the most trusted profession, nursing, is now filled with this career guide for nurses...written by a nurse FOR a nurse! The author will take you from hum drum to HOLD ON with insights on your nursing career!!! Motivation that every nurse needs to hear, and read." – Carmen Kosicek, RN, MSN; Author of '*Nurses, Jobs and Money -- A Guide to Advancing Your Nursing Career and Salary*'

"A wonderful read! Follow Elizabeth's great advice and it will move you toward the job – and life – you know is out there for you." – Connie Merritt, BSN, RN, PHN; Author of '*Too Busy for Your Own Good*'

"'*Your Next Shift*' will resonate with nurses that are looking for a change. Elizabeth Scala helps nurses strengthen their mindset, behaviors and motivations for the nurse entrepreneur adventure ahead!" –Michelle D. Podlesni, RN President- National Nurses in Business Association; Author of '*Unconventional Nurse: From Burnout to Bliss!*'

"Calling all disillusioned, disgruntled, or disenfranchised nurses! Elizabeth Scala has written a book for you that gives you the goods on how to find your passion in your work by shifting your mindset into an entrepreneurial mode. Get ready to rock your nursing practice!" – Lorry Schoenly, PhD, RN, CCHP-RN; Author of *'The Wizard of Oz Guide to Correctional Nursing'*

"*'Your Next Shift'* is a wonderful sequel to Elizabeth's first book: *'Nursing From Within: A Fresh Alternative to Putting Out Fires and Self-Care Workarounds'*. Elizabeth clearly writes in her own unique voice- and this makes her books enjoyably readable.

My key takeaways surround the idea of nurse entrepreneurial mindsets. Nurses are not traditionally trained to be business people. They may know what entrepreneurs are but may equate ownership to that ideal to rich business people featured in *Success Magazine*. Nurses are famous for their co-dependency. You might say transcending this one debilitating mindset is the great shining jewel of Elizabeth's wonderful books." –Kate Loving Shenk, BSN, RN; Author of *'The Prayer Prescription Series'*

"This book is a must-read for nursing students, new graduates and experienced nurses alike. If you're looking for practical tools and positive solutions to your nursing career challenges; then this is the book for you." –Caroline Porter Thomas; Author of *'New Nurse?: How to Get, Keep and LOVE Your First Nursing Job!'*

"Elizabeth Scala nailed it – literally! In *'Your Next Shift'*, she articulates what each of us, as nurses, has felt and experienced at one time or another in our professional careers. As one who never plans to quit working, I could easily relate to her concept of loving what you do, and doing it because you truly love it. A must read!" –Sharon M. Weinstein, MS, RN, CRNI, FACW, FAAN; Author of *'B is for Balance, 12 Steps Toward Having Balance at Home and at Work'*

"*'Your Next Shift'* provides an entrepreneurial toolset, which is applicable to any nursing specialty, for nurses who are struggling to find fulfillment and passion in their careers." –Brittney Wilson, BSN, RN; Author of *'The Nerdy Nurse's Guide to Technology'*

Well, Dad. This one's for you.
To my father: from Daddy's corvette show girl to all grown up nurse entrepreneur, I am forever grateful. As a man who has worked for decades as a hardworking professional you have taught me so much about work ethic, dedication, professionalism and accountability. My business would not be where it is today without the life lessons I have received from you. Thank you so much for teaching me about perseverance and commitment to getting the job done. My intention is to continue to make you proud... now let's start planning our Semester at Sea!

TABLE OF CONTENTS

Foreword
Preface
Acknowledgements

Introduction

    My Nursing Journey in Brief
    Loving Patient Care, Lacking in Self-Care
    Decision Time- *THE* Fork in the Road
    Expand Your Mind: New Skill-Sets from Beyond Nursing
    Learn Faster (From My Mistakes!)- To Receive Results
    Have Fun While You Read!

Part One: Background & Foundational Framework

CHAPTER 1: THE GAP ANALYSIS — **1**
    Start Where You're At to Move Yourself Forward
    Avoid the Perils and Pitfalls of Bright Shiny Objects
    De-Clutter the Mental Muck
    It's Time to Quit Playing Small
CHAPTER 2: MINDSET MATTERS MOST — **10**
    Case in Point: Scenarios from the People in Scrubs
    How to Tap into the Power of the Mind
    Which Mindset Mistakes Might You be Making?
CHAPTER 3: HOW TO THINK LIKE A SUCCESSFUL NURSE — **28**
    Feel the Lighter Energy Ahead
    Surround Yourself with Success
    How to Receive the Results You Crave
    Universal Laws Applied (In Nursing Practice)

Part Two: Nine Practical Applications for Your Nursing Career

CHAPTER 4: ENJOYMENT NOW BREEDS SUCCESS LATER — **46**
    The Topsy-Turvy World of a Nursing Career
    How to View Losing a Job as a Positive Experience
    Patience is Progress
CHAPTER 5: CLEARLY PLAN YOUR ROLE IN THE FUTURE — **53**
    Set Your Sights on the Future
    How to Attract the Nursing Career of Your Dreams
    Observe What Matters Most (Your Thoughts)
CHAPTER 6: TRUST IN THE PROCESS OF PATIENT FLOW — **58**
    How to Make What's 'Simple' Easy
    Tune In and Listen to the Signs
    Let Go of One Thing (And Open Up Doors to Your Future)
CHAPTER 7: SHIFT YOUR FOCUS — **64**
    Turning Values into Value
    Keep It Simple- Focus on What's In It for Them
    A Sure-Fire Way to Success (Solve Their Problem)

CHAPTER 8: KEEP GETTING THEIR ATTENTION   **69**
    Be Persistent... and Professional
    Follow Up: In a Way that Works
    Creativity, Connections and Continuity
CHAPTER 9: FEEL AND DO: KNOWLEDGE IS POWER   **75**
    Money, Money, Money! Master Your Numbers
    How to Face Your Fears
    Turn Your Power into Your Success
CHAPTER 10: CELEBRATE THE SMALL STUFF...
AND THE MIDDLE, BIG AND IN-BETWEEN!   **81**
    It's Perfectly OK (Even Necessary) to Toot Your Own Horn
    How to Keep Up with the Pace of Success
    What's the Point of Living if You're Not Learning?
CHAPTER 11: ASK FOR HELP WHETHER YOU'RE   **90**
    If You're Lost- You Need One Thing
    How to Get Exactly What You Want (And Need)
    Delegation Doesn't Only Happen in the Hospital
CHAPTER 12: IT'S OK TO BE YOU   **97**
    What to Do When You Throw Out All of Your Best Laid Plans
    Show Up in the Very Best Way that You Can
    Is it Passion? Or Profession? (Maybe a Little Bit of Both!)
CHAPTER 13: TYING IT ALL TOGETHER IN THE VERY BEST WAY   **103**
    Laughter is the Greatest Medicine of All
    Top Ten List: Entrepreneurial Tactic Recap

Part Three: Just for Today: A Step-By-Step Guide to Career Bliss

BONUS CHAPTER: 10 SIMPLE STEPS FOR NURSING CAREER JOY...
ON A DAILY BASIS!   **109**
    How to Do What I've Done (My Secret Sauce to Success)
    A Glimpse into the Life of Elizabeth Scala...
    Now Get Out There and Do It Yourself!

Appendix
About the Author
Up Close & Personal

FOREWORD

A shift change has needed to occur in nursing for many years now. These small paradigm shifts are in fact occurring on a micro level in our profession, and it's now time to bring our collective genius together to amplify our voices and elevate our thinking as a whole.

As a nurse and serial entrepreneur, I know that mindset is really at the core of one's own success. This concept has actually been vital to the success of my businesses. After seventeen years in various entrepreneurial endeavors ranging from small start-ups and side projects to large scale companies that went from grassroots to a global presence, I've taken quite a few emotional right hooks that would have likely collapsed just about anyone.

I've been fortunate enough however to appreciate a significantly higher number of successes than I did "opportunities." Now you might be telling yourself that I probably meant to say failures instead of opportunities, right? Well, I actually have no problem with saying failure. I'm just preparing you for that shift in mindset you are about to embark on.

To get vulnerable for a moment and for the sake of transparency I will share with you that I've definitely fallen hard in some of my business ventures. Whether it was picking the wrong business partner, not having enough start-up capital, or my overreliance on just a single concept that ultimately didn't reach the target market, it was actually mindset that fueled my desire to learn from these mistakes and rise up out of the ashes to begin again.

I can assure you that I take nothing for granted and I am proud to be considered a successful entrepreneur, but I've worked hard to get here. More importantly however is that I also take even more pride in being able to openly share my failures. These experiences are what have given me the expertise to help other entrepreneurs find their own success.

I have fallen, I have failed, and yes, it felt like I had been chewed up and spit back out. The thing is though is that I'm not afraid of failure or the word because I'm going to win every time. It just comes down to both my experience and ability to shift my mindset to embrace every failure as an opportunity for growth. Elizabeth Scala's *'Your Next Shift'* is going to help you discover this mindset on your own using the tips outlined in this very book.

Looking into the mirror isn't always pleasant. You may or may not like what you see. It is however a necessary rite of passage one must go through to better connect with oneself. If you are unable connect with yourself, then how can you authentically connect with your clients or those you're working with? I'll go ahead and remove the suspense and give you the answer now. You can't.

One of the best pieces of advice that I would have given you up until this moment is that you really need to go out and get this book. But, it seems as if you've already taken this next step at shifting your focus and you've made it this far into an abridged version of a spirited rant that I seem to be on, so I'll give you my next piece of advice. Anyone who has some skin in the game and willing to not only share their successes, but also to share their failures, fears and frustrations is someone I hold in very high regard. Elizabeth Scala IS this person and she is going to help guide you on this journey. You are not alone and she is with you right now, step-by-step.

Having known Elizabeth over these last few years is truly an honor and a gift for me, and I appreciate that our passion and purpose are aligned. You too will likely discover that *'Your Next Shift'* is purposefully written with you in mind.

My final piece of advice for you is that when someone is willing to become this transparent and this vulnerable, then it is best to do everything you can to mute the "noise," tear down the obstacles, and allow yourself to actually hear what is being shared. Listen to Elizabeth and also listen to yourself because it is going to matter and it will elevate your thinking in a way that will empower you to win every time, no matter the circumstances.

It's time to get comfortable with YOU and start connecting on a level that will have you living and working your full potential. Consider 'Your Next Shift' your gift to help you start this journey.

Now let's start blazing these trails together.

Kevin Ross, RN, BSN
Entrepreneur, Investor, Speaker, and Nurse

CEO and Founder of Spire Health Partners, Inc., Founder of Innovative Nurse and The Innovative Nurse Show, Co-Host and Founder at RN FM Radio, and champion of out of the box thinking.

PREFACE

One of the things I love about being a nurse entrepreneur is that I get to be the nurse I *want* to be. Anyone that knows me will tell you that I am very observant. I'm always watching. Listening. In big groups, I tend to sit off to the side and observe. One might view this as 'shy' or 'standoffish'. I like to think I am doing my 'homework'.

One perk of being my own boss is that my work is very flexible, very fluid. Those of you, who have been watching my evolution as a nurse entrepreneur, know that my business has changed in many ways since its inception. From the days of 'health and wellness' coaching with Living Sublime Wellness, to the RejuveNation Collaboration video summits; from speaking to writing- my work has shifted a lot over time.

This is the beauty of the nursing profession. We do not have to stay 'stuck' in one place. If, one day, we come to realize we are no longer happy with our current role, we can do something about it. We can change jobs, move to a new specialty, or even try out a new shift.

'*Your Next Shift*' is a culmination of all of the above. I observed the trends in nursing: listened to what was being discussed both on and offline in terms of job dissatisfaction, burnout and fatigue. I shifted the solutions I offer: instead of forcing health and wellness information; I have chosen to provide valuable resources that will help nurses enjoy their careers. Finally, after much reflection and market analysis, I bring you '*Your Next Shift*', which will provide you with innovative tools and out-of-the box thinking, to help you "level-up" your nursing career.

We all know that nursing is tough work. Gosh, I feel like I have said the previous sentence so many times that I am starting to sound like a broken record. Yet, it is important to point this out because with a difficult career comes obstacles, challenges and the occasional disappointment. Let me share a little secret with you: it doesn't have to be that way.

In nursing school (and beyond) we are taught clinical skills, problem-solving methods, theoretical frameworks and so much more. When we get out into the 'real world' we build on this knowledge with experience, thus enhancing our nursing expertise. What I have found is that while we as nurses are tremendously skilled at being a 'nurse'- we are less equipped to handle the complexity of our career as a whole.

We have book knowledge. We excel at clinical tasks. Yet, we need more. Whether consciously or unconsciously, we hit a certain career plateau which can cause us to feel stuck, bored or disgruntled in our nursing roles.

'Your Next Shift' offers solutions. Like you, I am also a nurse. So, I have received those skill sets required by the nursing profession just like you… and I have something more. Over the past several years, I have been building my business. I have learned from, studied with and been coached by, a lot of entrepreneurs. From marketing to sales, social media to in-person networking- I have seen (and continue to), heard and read it all.

And that's what I am here to share with you today. This book, *'Your Next Shift'*, is about bringing you an extra set of tools. I offer an additional skill set. It is time. It is time for you to "level-up" your nursing career from adequate to awesome.

Over the next several pages, I will share with you six of the critical mistakes every nurse needs to avoid. To counterbalance that, I will highlight the seven mindsets you absolutely need for success. I'll reveal my top entrepreneurial traits and teach you a step-by-step solution (that I used and continue to use on a daily basis) that will catapult your nursing career forward. Most importantly, you will learn how to think like an entrepreneur in your nursing practice… whether or not you ever want to become one.

That really is the best part of this entire book. It can work for you wherever you are as a nurse (or nursing student). You do not have to give up clinical practice and become a nurse entrepreneur to access the value in these methods. The entrepreneurial techniques discussed in this book have helped me become a better business woman, and more importantly, they have helped me grow as a human being.

I encourage you to read *Your Next Shift* in the way that serves you most. However, I will share with you my experience and what has worked for me when I read a book like this with an abundance of new techniques and information. Well, there are two ways that have worked for me really, but it all depends on how 'new' the content is to me.

If this material is totally foreign to you and you are not even sure it *'is'* for you- I suggest reading the book at your own pace, cover to cover. Allow yourself time to digest the material. This calls for some reflection and processing on a more global level. Then, after you have had some time to marinate on the concepts, take yourself through the book a second time, taking notes in whatever way works best for you.

On the other hand, if you're ready to dive right in- then do as I am doing with the book I am currently reading. I have a legal pad and pen in hand. I write in the margins, bunny ear the pages and take all sorts of notes to refer to later. This way, I ensure that I actually go back and implement what I have learned. I want the same for you: take what you read and do something with it. I am super excited to be of service as we begin to level-up your nursing career. Now let's get to it…

ACKNOWLEDGEMENTS

Special thanks to my editor, Ms. Scott. You can find out more about her work at www.facebook.com/payitforwardnow and www.facebook.com/360shapeup.

I want to give a very huge thank you to my cover designer, Joyce Fler Reyes, whose creative and professional work can be found at http://joyceflerdesigns.weebly.com.

To all of the pre-reviewers, the foreword author, Kevin Ross, and everyone who helped make this book rise to the top of the nursing profession- thank you so much.

I also want to acknowledge the people of Create Space, Amazon's Self-Publishing arm, which makes it really easy, fun and flexible to get my work out there.

Thank you to Peter Bowerman (who doesn't even know me and probably never will). Your book, The Well-Fed Self-Publisher, was like a bible to me as I wrote, published and continue to market this book (and all of my books, really).

A very special thank you goes out to not only my business coach, Alicia Forest, but to all of the OBBW'ers who helped me along with title suggestions, launch ideas and love and continued support.

To my husband, Drew. Thank you for being continuously overjoyed by my success and allowing me to live my life with passion, joy and fun.

To nurses everywhere. Acute care, academia, clinics, outpatient centers, retirees, nursing students… Thank you from the bottom of my heart. You are my inspiration. You are my muse. You are the reason I continue to write.

INTRODUCTION

I want to start out by saying this right up front. In no way, shape or form is this book about getting nurses to leave their clinical roles. I actually went back and forth a *LOT* on how to write it; whether I should; or if I even *could* write this book.

The reason I struggled so much is simple: I never want to encourage nurses to leave the bedside. That is not what my work is all about. In fact, when I started out as a nurse entrepreneur and was developing my 'elevator pitch' to my 'target market' (things my coaches made me do to get clear on what my business was all about), I used to say something like this:

"I help nurses feel happier and healthier so that they don't have to leave the bedside."

Why was I so adamant about this? Well, to be honest with you, I really did not want to leave my clinical role. In '*Nursing from Within: A Fresh Alternative to Putting Out Fires and Self-Care Workarounds*', I wrote about my journey from 'hell to health'. In my keynote speeches, workshops and webinars I always introduce myself with 'my journey to well-being'.

Yes, I left psychiatric nursing. Yes, I had to do it for my own sanity and self-care. No, I really *did not* want to leave patient care. And yes, I do miss it all of the time. In fact, so much so, that at the time of this writing I often thought about going back and still even search out job openings in psychiatry from time-to-time.

So, I want to be really, really clear about this right up front. My intention has never been (and will never be) to sway nurses away from roles in direct patient care. There is no way that each and every one of us can leave our jobs and become entrepreneurs. Trust me, it is not for everyone. (I even question what the heck I am doing now and then!)

OK, phew. Just wanted to get that off of my chest. Now, moving onto bigger and better things... Introducing you to what this book is all about.

A Special Place in My Heart

As I mentioned above, I was a psychiatric nurse and if this is the first time you are finding me, then you may or may not know all about my history of leaving that job to go work part-time at a wellness center, running a physician referred exercise program. Well I did that.

In 2009, I made a very difficult decision. I left my safe and secure full-time job to go monitor beginning, out of habit, or those exercisers who needed special assistance. Trust me; this was a huge risk. So much so, that when I called my parents, I literally left a voicemail: *"I'm leaving my job. Bye!"* Not only was this decision dicey, terrifying and fun all at the same time, but it was hard.

Guess what I loved most about my psych job? You got it. The patients. Before I became a nurse, I actually graduated with a degree in psychology and a minor in sociology. I don't know what it is about me, but people with mental illness just have a special place in my heart. Maybe it is my family history of alcoholism and depression. Maybe it's all of those criminal type shows I enjoy. Or, maybe the fact that I love to do jigsaw puzzles, frame them and hang them all around my house. Who knows? But, I loved being on the psych floor.

Don't Do What I Did

So, in 2010, I was out of there. That winter, during one of Baltimore's biggest back-to-back blizzards of all time, I worked my last weekend shift (yes!) and after a lovely two week vacation, I reported to my new job at the gym.

You might be wondering (if you don't know me at all, yet) - how come you left the psych job if you loved the patients so much? Great question!

This answer is sort of lengthy, so I'll do my best to be succinct (not one of my bigger strengths). The reason back then (in 2009) was: I was miserable. Inside and out; I was a wreck. I took no care of my own well-being and I was sick and tired of being… well, sick and tired. I also had a very nasty perspective on life. I blamed *everyone* else but me for all of my pain.

It was my manager's fault and the assistant manager for not assisting her. The staff on my unit was to blame. Heck, the entire organization was at fault. I pointed fingers, spread gossip and was an all out Bi-otch (excuse my language).

The second part of this answer comes in the here-and-now. Because of all of the materials I am about to share with you in this book (ooh, a reason to keep on reading!), I have since let all of those harsh feelings, judgments and negativity go. In fact, I have visited my old unit and really enjoyed it. I have taught Reiki and shared Reiki with several of my ex-coworkers. I feel absolutely no ill will to the staff, unit or department.

And here's why: it was all me.

It was my perspective of how things were. It was my own lack of self-care. It was the fact that I had no coping skills, took part in absolutely no spiritual practice and did nothing to better myself or my mindset. So, I did what I don't want any of you to do.

I ran.

I left the job on the psych floor, even though I loved the patients, because I was running away from a job I no longer enjoyed. While I do encourage you to work in a career you love; leaving a job because you don't like it without any thought of what you *do* want to do with your life instead is no way to change your circumstances.

The Fork in Your Road

OK, so I bet we need some clarity here. You might be reading and thinking to yourself, *'On the one hand she wants me to enjoy my work; on the other, she is telling me not to leave my job. I'm confused. What the heck is she talking about?'*

Awesome question (and great insight into the fact that I am sort of contradicting myself here). So, let me clear this up for you. I present on this topic in one of my webinars entitled, *'Create Career Resilience for Self'*, and so I am getting a visual from one of the Power Point slides in my head as I type these words.

The way I see it is, with respect to your career, you can come to a fork in the road. You may totally enjoy your career and think to yourself, *'This book is not for me. I am happy with where I am.'* On the other hand, you may know that you are unhappy and at the same time know that there is nothing else you want to do in terms of your work (think about my above example of loving my psych patients). In this case, you feel stuck. As if nothing will ever change or get better. That is an uncomfortable place to be; I hear you.

The final place you may reside (well, there are tons of options, but for today's sake let's just look at these three) is totally unhappy and ready to make a change. Woo hoo! I love it. Now, here is where I caution you: make a change based on what you *do* want instead of what you don't want. (No worries about fully understanding this concept; more on it later in the pages to follow.)

All I am suggesting is this: you can find yourself in any old place in terms of your nursing career and there is always room for growth. Hence, the nature of this book: moving ourselves from adequate to awesome in the way we think, feel and experience our job. This may mean becoming a nurse entrepreneur. Or, it may not. It's whatever you decide. The best thing is that the information and resources laid out in this book can help you wherever you are at.

Not sure you trust me? Let me lay out an overview of what we'll cover in '*Your Next Shift*'.

Why this Book?

There are some really great books out there on a whole host of topics that might be similar to this book. Trust me, I did the research. There are books teaching nurses how to enjoy their careers, books on becoming nurse entrepreneurs, and books on career strategies in nursing. Books on interviewing, resumes and what to do when you are fresh out of nursing school. Gosh, if you want to find a book on any certain topic- in today's day and age- I bet you can. (See the appendix for books I recommend.)

So, what does '*Your Next Shift*' offer that others don't? A lot. Here are several of the key highlights that make this book an awesome choice for those of you looking to level-up your careers:

1. Entrepreneurial Techniques

As I mentioned in previous pages, this book adds to our nursing backgrounds. Sure, we have the clinical skills and specialty knowledge, but what about that added boost that you're looking for in your career? Continuing to learn more '*nursing*' skills may or may not be the way to enhance your particular career. I guess that keeping up with technology and learning about the new machines on your unit is important, but what about those of us who are looking to be cutting edge?

In this book, I will touch on some key concepts that every successful solo-preneur applies. Things like knowing your numbers to being consistent with your follow up. From your unique selling position to serving with solutions. Again, those of you reading who may not have any interest in being a nurse entrepreneur; that's totally cool! You can absolutely apply what you will read in this book to your nursing career, without leaving patient care.

2. Learn from Example

I don't know about you, but I like to learn by modeling what I read and hear. I learn from example. Actually, getting my hands on the material and doing it in action.

Well, that's how I am going to teach you in this book. When we get to the section that teaches the ten entrepreneurial action items, I am literally going to be sharing from my own lessons learned.

In fact, I went back to my old coaching groups (I had my coach give me access to pages from years ago) and re-read all of my posts. I then took clips of my process (the good, bad and the ugly) and will be sharing them here with you, word-for-word so that you can get a feel for how I learned these lessons in that very moment. Then, you can learn from example as we go through the contents of this book together.

3. A Focus on Process and Outcome

Many books focus on the process- how to do the steps being taught to the reader. While I enjoy that and agree that we need process to move us forward, let's be honest; we want results! And if you're reading this book, then part of me can assume that you are looking for some outcomes related to your nursing career.

Building upon what I said in number two, I know that what I am sharing with you delivers outcomes. How do I know that? I do these exercises, especially the ones I will teach you in the ten step system (see bonus chapter), on a daily basis. Trust me; if I miss several days of doing these exercises in a row- I feel it. I notice I don't experience the same 'results' in my business when I am out of practice. More on this later...

4. A Really, Really Fun Book

Those of you who are reading may or may not know that my number one value is FUN. In my previous book, '*Nursing from Within*',

I covered a four-step process to uncovering your true heart's desires. Your values, in essence. So since 'fun' is my absolute number one- the thing I hold in the highest regard (and don't judge me, we all have our unique value system) - you can definitely count on this also being a really fun book.

There will be no stuffy, academic writing here. In fact, when I get my books edited I have to find a proof-reader who will let me keep my own 'voice' since I know I am breaking every single grammar rule known to man and that's what makes this (and all of my) book(s) fun. I hope that you find the reading easy, conversational and upbeat. The point is to actually get through the entire book, right?

5. An Innovative Solution

I like to think of myself as a pioneer, a visionary really. What I am doing with this book (and most of my work, really) is applying concepts from other arenas to the nursing landscape. So again, to borrow from 'Nursing from Within' one more time, that book pulled theories from universal law, energy principles and spiritual practice to teach concepts that nurses could use to make those inner shifts so that they could more fully enjoy their external environments.

This book is no different. I am taking ideas from the entrepreneurial environment and applying them to our nursing careers in hopes of teaching concepts that will allow for more joy, satisfaction and resilience in nursing practice. In fact, I'll go out on a limb here and boldly say: my intention is that this book offers you solutions to your nursing career problems. So much so, that after you read this book (and implement the processes), your job will never feel like work again.

It's true. We can all live our passion in our work (see the Appendix for more resources on this). And through some entrepreneur mindset shifts, we can totally rock our nursing practice. So who's with me? Let's do this...

Part One

Chapter 1
The Gap Analysis

Warning: this first chapter may feel a little uncomfortable. In fact, I am starting out with something that isn't very typical of me. I'm beginning our journey together with what could potentially be 'wrong' with our careers. Why is this unlike me? In short, I am a firm believer in what Carl Jung once said:

"What we resist, persists."

However, in order to move ourselves forward, I also believe that we have to know where we are starting. In working with several coaches over the years, I have come to notice that many of us use one single method in all of our work: the gap analysis.

Any good coach will certainly do one thing: get you to realize where you are at. Then, they will take you through a variety of exercises that will highlight where you want to be and then, (here's the kicker of how they get you to sign on to work with them… and it's OK I am sharing this with you, since it's no secret. I do it too.) they get you to see what it will take to move you from where you are at (point A in the here-and-now) to point B (where you'd like to be).

So, the paragraphs above are my quick disclaimer. They're also a way for me to point out that what we'll cover in this chapter may not be the most 'fun', but I can assure you, after we get through this part, we'll never come back to doom and gloom again.

A Multifaceted Approach

If you've read 'Nursing from Within: A Fresh Alternative to Putting Out Fires and Self-Care Workarounds', you know that I started out in a similar fashion. I highlighted the various issues that come up in our nursing practice and broke them into three categories: self, others and global challenges. What follows here is comparable.

I'd like to start off by highlighting some of our nursing career obstacles. Some have to do with our own selves and the mindsets we bring to our work, while others are purely job related and may be beyond our individual control. This is all to show us that there certainly are reasons for our discomfort, but the good news is: some we can also choose to change.

An Overwhelming System

Let's start out this time on a global scale. Healthcare, as we know it, is shifting. It continues to change. Couple that with uncertainty in our economy, world health crises, and the age of digital information and it's no wonder we feel fatigued.

One of the reasons you may have found yourself unhappy with your job is because being an actual nurse gets harder and harder each day. You may feel like you don't have enough time to be with your patients. You might worry that you're missing crucial information. You start to rush around from task-to-task, feeling a little bit like a chicken with its head cut off. You think to yourself, 'This isn't why I went into nursing or how I thought my career would be'.

Plain and simple: it's tough to be a nurse these days. We want to be present with our patients and provide good care, yet our j-o-b gets in the way. Let's be blunt: maybe you're just not that happy being a nurse anymore because you actually feel like your job doesn't let you be one!

What I've just described deals with some overarching issues that are beyond our control. So, what happens when we feel like our lives are out of control? That we can't impact change? That we can't be heard? We feel terrible. Be honest. It feels really, really bad to be 'told' what to do. To be talked 'down' to. To be impressed upon.

We spend a large majority of our lives at work. So, we want to go there and actually enjoy ourselves, right? We want to feel as if our job made an impact. That our work was meaningful!

If you find yourself in this bucket- totally disgruntled with the entire system- then maybe it is time for a change for you. I can't be the one to tell you that. But, I encourage you to keep on reading because my hope is that you find the solutions you are looking for. OK, so we tackled the 'global' challenges of being a nurse. Let's get into some more of the nitty-gritty, self-imposed obstacles.

Lost in the Crowd

Woops. There is one other area to touch on before we get to the mindset piece. It's the notion of distraction.

So above, I alluded to the digital age of information. Well, this is compounded by the fact that many of us are also out of spiritual touch with life. I'm not talking about 'religion'. In fact, I received feedback on my previous book, 'Nursing from Within', that a nurse could not offer an endorsement of the book because of my 'religious' beliefs. Let me share a little secret with you: I'm not a 'religious' person. Spirituality is not the same thing as religion. At all.

OK. Let me get down from my soap box here. But really, with this age of digital information comes a very high likelihood that you will encounter distraction and if you don't have a spiritual practice to bring you back into the here-and-now, you're at much greater risk for getting lost in the crowd.

Besides the constant and all-encompassing distractions, we are also faced with the busy-ness of life. I don't mean taking care of 'business'. I literally mean being busy all of the time. Busy because of helping others. Busy because of work, family and friends. Busy for the sake of being busy. Busy work to simply distract us from the dissatisfaction we feel from it all. Busy to deter us from making any changes. Busy 'doing' to avoid 'being'. (Hence, more need for spiritual practice.)

Even if you're not that 'busy', you may experience 'bright shiny object' syndrome in terms of your career, which even further prevents you from enjoying your work. 'What is 'bright shiny object' syndrome?' you might ask? Great question.

Bright shiny object syndrome is what happens when we feel compelled to do things we see others succeeding at. Think of nursing for a second. How many letters do you have after your name? How many degrees have you received? Do you have a specialty certification? Are you getting certified in something else that is non-nursing?

Don't get me wrong. Education is a great thing and I've certainly fallen victim to 'bright shiny object' syndrome. I've got my masters degrees in nursing and business, but have I ever used them? Not really. I am certified in not one, but two health and wellness coaching programs. Do I actually 'coach' clients? Not anymore.

On a larger scale, what I am referring to here is being inauthentic. Part of the reason we may find ourselves no longer enjoying our careers as much as we could be is because we are doing what everybody else has done.

We see a colleague go back to school and think to ourselves: 'Maybe I need to get another degree'. We hear of a neighbor taking a certification in a holistic practice, and before we even do any research to see if it's for us, we sign up for the course. I'm not saying everyone does this with every decision, but ask yourself: am I trying to be someone that I am not?

One reason we may find ourselves stuck, disgruntled or even fatigued by our nursing careers is that we are no longer using our unique gifts. Our individual talents have become stifled. We are so influenced by others and what we see them doing all day long; we've forgotten how to be ourselves. It's one thing to be part of a group (the nursing profession); it's another to fall victim of group thinking.

Monkey Mind

Alright, now here is where we get into self-sabotage. Don't worry- after this next section; we are moving on to brighter pastures so stick with me for a little bit longer.

The first self-imposed obstacle is one I shared with you in the introduction portion of this book. One I did very well. One I have quite a bit of experience with. It's that catastrophic thinking. That person (it was me!) who blames everything and everyone else for the problems around them.

This mindset includes thoughts like this: 'Things will never change'. Or 'It's everybody's fault'. Worst yet: 'My luck is terrible'. One might even view this type of all-or-nothing thinking as playing the role of the victim. 'We' can't do anything about our situation so it must be everyone else around that must be out to get us.

Again, I'm the last one to point fingers. That was me. I was THE Negative Nancy Nurse. I take full ownership of this and I'm here to tell you with absolute enthusiasm, if this is you, don't worry. You too can change. (This book can be your first step.)

Another caveat we are faced with is our own mind. On the one hand, we love the mind, right? It helps us think, remember, talk, move, achieve and excel in life. We need our minds in order to do everything and anything we want to do each day. On the other, our minds can lead to our entire downfall.

Have you ever heard that our greatest asset can also be our biggest challenge? Well, in this case, that is what the mind can be. We can use the great power of our mind to lift ourselves up, enjoy our careers and live a totally exceptional life. Or, as we saw in the previous paragraphs about catastrophic thinking, our minds can totally get in our way.

And guess what? I know you know this, but have you really 'thought' about it? Our minds never stop. Ever. Try not to think. What happens? You immediately start thinking of something. That or you realize that you were deeply lost in thought. Unconscious thought that you were not even aware of!

Even as you are reading the words on this page -in this paragraph, -in this sentence… are you fully present and aware? Or is your mind distracted, off somewhere else?

If we are unconscious of our thoughts, we can fall victim to a 'monkey mindset'. This refers to the broken record of worry. Again, our minds never stop and one thing they may be doing all day is worrying nonstop. Worried if we will get to work on time. Worried who we are working with. Worried about our assignment. Worried if we can leave on time. Worry, worry, and constant worry… all day long.

It doesn't just have to be worry, my friend. It can be fear. It can be doubt. It can be criticism that's self-inflicted. My point is, if you are unaware of your thoughts, there is a very good chance they are running your life and more often than not, in a negative way. In a way that can lead to career dissatisfaction and disengagement with life.

OK, almost done, I promise. The final self-inflicted barrier comes from what I mentioned above in terms of self-imposed criticism. We put ourselves down. We second guess our success. We think to ourselves: 'I'll never be good enough to get, be, reach…'

So we remain stuck. Especially in our careers. We don't take chances and never make changes to move ourselves forward. Sure, being unhappy in our jobs is no fun, but it's a lot easier than making a change. Sometimes the effort required to do something different is so daunting that we'd rather stay miserable where we are at. What do we do then? Refer to the above on distraction. We distract ourselves in other ways so that we can 'get through' the work day.

Time for a Change

Well this is it. We've come to our crossroads. It is time for you to make a decision. If you think you want to stay exactly where you are, then there is no reason for you to continue reading this book (my goodness, did I just say that?).

But, if you're ready to say 'YES'; if you're ready for a change, ready to quit playing it small. Then come right along, my friend. Because what's to come is so very exciting. Let's get to the shifts, innovations and solutions that will have you enjoying your nursing career for years to come. Here we go!

Chapter 2
Mindset Matters Most

What I'm about to share with you is no secret. You may have even heard it before. In fact, you may even believe it. Yet, it's so super-duper important I could not leave it out of a book like this. You ready? Here it is…

Mindset is everything.

In terms of career enjoyment, quality of life, outlook on relationships and even money, income and wealth- mindset matters. The most. There is no way to get around this. Your mindset is everything.

Now, I don't want to take up a ton of real estate in this book going through the background on how mindset impacts everything (you can check out '*Nursing from Within*' for more information on that), but what I will do is offer the following two scenarios as a teachable moment…

Scenario One

Say you're driving to work in the morning, all set for your day. You take this same route over and over again. Day in and day out; you could travel these roads in your sleep. So, it's no surprise that once in a while, while driving, your mind starts to wander. Today, you find yourself contemplating what the day ahead will bring…

The past two weeks on your nursing unit have been hell. Literally. There is a patient in room 311 who won't stop screaming; the team can't seem to get her medication regimen altered in such a way that doesn't make her delirious. You've been short staffed because there is a flu bug going around. The mandatory overtime has been off the charts and you feel like you've been living at your job. Between being at work, driving to work and sleeping a bit in between, everything these past two weeks has been totally and completely about your J-O-B.

So, as you are taking the commute into work, you lose yourself in your thoughts: *'Is it going to be another horrid day? What type of staffing will we have? Will I have time to go to the bathroom? Gosh, I better inhale this breakfast bar now… don't know when I'll get to eat. Better not drink too much coffee… Am I going to have to stay late again? Who will pick the kids up from school? Who will make dinner tonight? Oh heck; let's be honest. Take-out is so much easier…'*

The thoughts go on and on, almost never-ending. Then, all of a sudden a car in front of you stops short. You lay on your horn, feeling completely irritated. No, let's be honest. You're pissed. Now that you're shaken back to reality, you realize that you actually don't feel so good. When you really stop to think about it, you feel angry. Tired. Fed up. Full of frustration.

By the time you get into work you are so full of negativity it's no wonder that you snap at the new nursing student that you've been tasked to orient. *'Gosh, I didn't mean to be that rude,'* you shamefully think to yourself and thus, it continues as now you have that guilt to add to your list of bad feelings…

Scenario Two

Well, by no miracle at all you managed to get out of the unit on time today. Evening shift was fully staffed and you left right on schedule. As you walk to the car, you check your cell phone. *'Oh, what's this? My husband called. Let me listen to this voicemail…'*

You almost drop the phone. In total shock you play the message again, *'Honey, I got a sitter for the kids. I am taking you out to eat tonight. You've been working so hard; you deserve it. Meet me at Outback at 5 o'clock.'*

Sitting in the car, you are brought to tears. How wonderful this is. A night out on the town! But how tired I am; will I be much company for him?

You get to the restaurant, kiss your honey and are shown to your table. He is jabbering on about his day and you can't hear a thing. You're thinking about work: *'Did I pass along in report about that PRN I gave? Oh gosh, did I get Mr. Jones off of the commode?'* The waitress comes along and starts telling you about the specials and that's when you all about lose it. Or do you?

This waitress is nothing like you've seen before. She is over-the-top happy; full of pleasant conversation. She asks you and your husband questions about your interests, tells you about the best specials they have at the restaurant and even gives you ideas about other places to find really good meal deals. '*Is she for real?*' you think to yourself. '*Why is she being* so *nice?*'

At first, her joyful demeanor pisses you off and you even tell your husband that. Her smile is getting under your skin. Her silly laugh is making your stomach turn. What the heck is she so darn happy about?

Then, something strange happens; you notice you are feeling a little bit better than when you entered the restaurant. You are finding it easier to focus on your husband and his conversation about the kids. You realize your mood is lifting and you are feeling, dare you say it, happy?

Brainwashed By Our Thoughts

What happened in the two polarizing scenarios above? Well, each of the two stories highlighted the very fact that our thoughts influence how we feel. We were introduced to mindset and the very way it can impact our day.

Let me ask you a question: Have you ever tried subliminal messages? You know those messages that get put into music, background noise or melodic sounds?

I first heard of them on that eighties show I used to love, 'Saved by the Bell'. The main character, Zack Morris, put them into some cassette tapes he gave to the one he lusted over in almost every episode, Kelly Kapowski. In fact, he shared them with his best friend 'Screech' and they both tried to brainwash the girls into saying 'yes' to dates for the Valentine's Day dance. Well, in the end, they wound up getting caught- but before that- the tapes actually *did* work.

Why was this? Well, the answer is simple. Subliminal messages are processes that you may not even be aware of. They are literally below the threshold of your conscious mind. Specific regions of the brain are activated, without our knowledge. In fact, I've started to try them out in terms of increasing my self-confidence and money mindset just this past month. I'm not sure yet of the results, since I just started using them, but I'll let you know.

This next chapter will take us through some of the mindset perils. First, I will cover the six critical mindset mistakes every nurse needs to avoid making and don't worry, I am sure you're out there thinking: '*I thought that you said the last chapter was the final* 'gloom and doom'*portion of this book*'. Well, yes. It most certainly was. However, I would be doing you a great disservice if I didn't cover how to steer clear of these mindset pitfalls.

To counterbalance the mindset mistakes, we will then journey through seven mindsets that will set you up for continued success in your nursing career. I am really looking forward to this part of the book (as you ought to be too) since these are the mindsets that really can change everything. OK, enough talking about these things. Let's get into action. Have your paper and pencil ready? Let's do this…

Mindset Mistakes

In a moment I am going to share a list of six top mindset mistakes. I tell you this right up front for a couple of reasons. The first is that I am sure there are many, many more mindset mistakes you and I might make in our lifetimes, but at the time of this writing I share with you the most common ones that many of us struggle with (raising my hand here, as I too have overcome many of these).

Another reason I share this with you right up front is this: be gentle with the material. Try to avoid putting up the defensive with immediate '*that's not me*' thinking. Be open to what's on this list and take honest inventory to see if any of these are challenging you. While this list may or may not be exhaustive, take time to honestly contemplate these monkey mindsets. The first step to making any change is having the awareness that we need to in the first place.

Here is my list of top six mindset mistakes to avoid (and then we'll take each of them in turn, one-by-one):

Fear
Doubt
Worry
Criticism

Lack Mentality
Negativity

Good. Get that list out of the way, right up front. Deal with it immediately so that we can move on to greener pastures, so to speak. Now, let's touch on each of these in brief so that in the chapters that follow we are free to offer up some solutions.

Stifling Rejection

Fear is probably one of the most debilitating mindsets of all. Fear can absolutely paralyze you from moving forward. If you are afraid of being rejected, becoming a failure or hearing the word 'no' you may never put yourself out there in a way that will "level-up" your career. Fear is probably the one that I struggled with the most.

High school was a really, really hard time for me.

From the very first day, it was full of disappointment and rejection. My best friend for close to eight years and I were finally 'there'. The big school. Changing classes. No more uniforms. Surrounded by a lot more people. This was going to be an awesome time for us... or so I thought. I guess she had other plans in mind.

It started off almost immediately. Her sister was older than us, I think maybe three years ahead of our grade, so my best friend from grammar and middle school was 'known' by the older, cooler kids. She had loads of new friends. Even boys started asking her out on dates. By the first winter, we were no longer 'best' friends. I felt she had totally dropped me as a friend, like I didn't even exist.

Then there was dating, boys and school events. Prom time was the worst. No one asked me to the dance. I heard through the grapevine that my classmates were trying to get this one boy to ask me to the Prom and he said he'd rather go alone. I never had a boyfriend in high school, not even close to one.

Finally, there was my senior year. The worst of it all. While losing my best friend from grade school was really tough, it did open me up to some new friends throughout high school. Or, again (are we sensing a pattern here?), so I thought. My senior year, me and my two 'best friends' went on a trip to the beach and ended up having a big old fight and the car ride home was spent in awkward silence. As my friend left me in my driveway, she rolled down her window to tell me that I was now cut out of their lives and would no longer be considered a friend to them.

Think I've been rejected once or twice? You bet…

Well, fast forward about fifteen years to the here-and-now. How did this fear of rejection impact me in my career? As a nurse entrepreneur, in more ways than one! From the fear of approaching others, to the fear of hearing a 'no' from potential clients; from the fear of making an offer to the fear of putting myself out there- I was afraid of everything.

Afraid of being a failure. Afraid people wouldn't like me. Afraid that they might realize I don't know it all or have all of the answers. What are you afraid of? Has fear-based thinking gotten in the way of your own career success?

Another interesting thing to mention here, which I will cover in more detail in later chapters, is this notion of unfounded fears. So what are you afraid of *AND* is there really a reason to be scared? I'll give you a brief example.

Last week I was nervous. I was worrying about having enough money in my bank account (more on money issues in upcoming pages) to cover a large bill that was going to go through. My husband and I added a security system to our home (that's right; no more breaking in, you guys. LOL). Well, the installing technician told me that in about thirty days the balance of the bill would just be taken out of my account.

So, the time was getting close to when the extra $397.00 would be deducted from my bank account (I had paid cash at installation time). That same week some other stuff was coming out of my checking account and due to renting a moving truck and some additional expenses that were unusual for us; my husband and I were running low on cash.

It was on my mind all of the time. I'd walk up my driveway from walking my dog and start doing the math in my head, counting the days back from security system installation until the current date. I'd wake up in the morning before the alarm, doing the bills and numbers in my head. Finally, it dawned on me. I could eliminate all of this fear.

I called the security system and just asked them: '*What date will this balance go through?*' The woman was extremely helpful and friendly. She calmed my fears that the remaining charge wouldn't be drawn out until after my husband and I got paid on Friday. Phew!

I was feeling all of this fear for nothing. No reason at all. So, I encourage you to do the same with some of your fears. Here's an exercise for you to try on your own. Write down each of your fears on a piece of paper. One by one, list them out. Yes, I am aware that it may not be that much fun. Yet here's the great part. Take each one and really be honest with yourself. Ask yourself: '*Is this fear real? Or is this an unfounded fear, based on no part of reality?*'

One of my very first coaches had me do this exercise with her and it really, really worked. She even added an extra caveat, which you can try too, if you like. Once you have your list of fears and your opinions on real versus unproven, ask someone else. A loved one. A close friend. Have a gentle, yet honest conversation with someone you hold in high regard and trust very much. Ask them. They have no skin in the game and are likely to give you their honest opinion.

Uncertainty Can Hold You Back

Let's move onto the next mistaken mindset we want to avoid: DOUBT. Now doubt can be just as debilitating, if not more so, than fear. Doubt has the capacity to completely paralyze you. On top of that, you can doubt so many things… many of which may impact your career.

One of the hardest things for any human being to do is to know their own worth. Their value. Sure, it's easy to praise, compliment and love another human being. But, what about ourselves? Especially us nurses. We can give a compliment, share praise and offer credit where credit is due. Yet, when it comes to turning that attention on ourselves, well goodness sakes, no one wants to come across as conceited, right?

There are other areas in your career you may be experiencing doubt. Do you doubt your ability to succeed? Doubt the chances you have to move up in your clinical ladder? Doubt that you are the right person for the job? Have you ever doubted the success of your work, second-guessed your expert opinion in the eyes of colleagues?

If you're thinking about becoming a nurse entrepreneur, doubt can severely limit your chances of success. If you don't value yourself or your message (which ultimately will become your product or service), how will you make money? If you don't see yourself as worthy of receiving clients, income or even success- how will you be able to stay in business?

Disbelieving and distrusting in your own abilities can definitely impact your achievements. Fear no more my friend. We will certainly cover this in upcoming chapters as we travel through methods of mindset shifts together.

Rumination Procrastination

Yikes, this list gets harder and harder by the minute. I know I said 'fear' was my largest hurdle to overcome, yet coming up on 'worry' I'm not so sure. Worry can completely consume you (and I), leaving us stuck in inaction.

In chapter seven of '*Nursing from Within*' I shared a wonderful little resource that I'd like to introduce here as well. It's just that important. Ready for this surefire way past all of the worries that have ever plagued you? Here it is: live in the here-and-now.

'Just for today' is a mantra I use over and over in my life. The rooms of Alcoholics Anonymous are also known for a similar line: *one day at a time.*

Worry is about living in the past. It's about ruminating over the future. It's being obsessed with things that are beyond our control. Things that may never even come to fruition. Worry is a tailspin. A rabbit hole that, if you're not aware of it, you can get very, very lost in.

'What if my big idea doesn't work? What if my product offer falls flat on its face? What if I can't make any money? What if? What if? What if?'

Gosh, even typing the above worries has me worried that if I worry in that way, it will bring me more worry. That I may never reach the life of my dreams. Enjoy lasting abundance. On and on and on… you get the picture!

Let's get past this worry before we all make ourselves crazy. Moving onto the next mindset to avoid… and don't worry (pun intended)- I'll definitely be sharing resources in the upcoming chapters that will help us all break free from the chains of fretful overwhelm.

Judge Much?

I don't mean others. While criticizing other people is never nice, here, we are talking about those judgments that are self-inflicted.

Does any of this sound familiar?

I'm not good enough.

I'm not smart enough.

I don't have enough experience.

I didn't do a good job.

I will always fail.

I'm stupid.

Talk like that to ourselves and it's no wonder we are, at best, floundering in our careers and yes, these are quite the extreme. I do agree, many of us are not saying these things to ourselves out loud.

But, honestly, what is your self-talk like? Do you put yourself down? Beat yourself up? Judge yourself too harshly?

In terms of being a nurse entrepreneur, you are going to have to put yourself out there (more on this later). In fact, any type of nurse these days is probably going to have to put him or herself out there and what I mean by "out there" is this: out in front of people. Out in public. Out on the 'big stage'.

Think about it: as a nurse entrepreneur, you are going to have to market and sell your business. But guess what? Even those non-nurse entrepreneurs out there, if you are a nurse looking for a new clinical role or job change of any kind, what will you have to do? Interview. Get in front of the prospective new manager, HR people or those that will be involved with giving you that new job.

Ralph Waldo Emerson once said: "A man is what he thinks about all day". Think we're not good enough or don't deserve that new job, guess what? We probably aren't going to get it. Why is that? Well, as I cover in many of my keynote presentations and webinar courses, everything is energy. Even that thought of '*I'm not good enough*' becomes an energetic frequency which people pick up on.

People can sense your energy. They will feel your vibration. So, if you are vibrating at a very self-critical frequency, you will literally emit that onto others and they will feel that from you.

There's Never Enough

Lack mentality can literally destroy our careers. Because of everything we have mentioned above (the power of thought, the energy of vibrations, etc.) I don't have much more to add on this mistaken mindset.

In the nursing world, we often struggle with lack mentality and focus on it. I am constantly hearing things like: '*We don't have enough resources. There isn't enough time. We don't have the staff.*' You get the idea.

While I am not downplaying the challenging environment of today's healthcare field, let me again remind you: what you think about you bring about; what you resist grows stronger. As Buddha once said, "All that we are is a result of what we have thought".

In essence, lack mentality is actually an accumulation of all of the things we have discussed thus far. It's a mindset of fear and worry. It's a feeling of doubt in the self. It's being critical of what's going wrong.

In terms of your nursing career, you've got to shift the focus from lack to abundance. While this may be difficult to do (which is OK, since this book is here to help you), it is the only way to make sustainable shifts in your professional role. Especially those of us, who want to change careers, do something different or even go into business for ourselves.

Lack mentality just has no place in the entrepreneurial world. In fact, it has no place in the professional world at all. Period. We live in an abundant and supporting universe. There is plenty for all of us. Here's a perfect example for you from the 'real world' space of health and wellness coaching.

As I shared in the introduction section of this book, I am actually certified as a health and wellness coach. In the early days of my business, I used to coach one-on-one clients around their holistic well-being. That meant working on anything from stress reduction to healthy eating, from getting more exercise to finding time and space for rejuvenation in one's busy life.

Well when I started out, coaching nurses on their health, I thought I had a very novel idea. Boy, a health and wellness coach for the nursing profession- people are going to be beating down my door! I mean there are over three million of us in the United State alone. Talk about a never-ending supply of potential clients. Right? Wrong.

When I entered the virtual space of an online business I was shocked into reality. There were health and wellness coaches all over the place. What was even worse? There were people who specialized in coaching nurses. My heart sank. No one's going to want to work with me, right? Wrong again!

What I didn't realize at that time, yet have come to realize since then, is that I am a unique individual. I show up as a coach in my own way. I am very different than how you may present yourself as a coach and you are very different than how the next person may offer their coaching style.

We are all individual beings with a distinct approach. What resonates with some people (which may or may not be my method) won't resonate with all people and that's great because then I can refer those potential clients out to you. Say a client comes to you, asking for help in an area that you don't specialize in. Guess what? Yep! You can send them right over to me.

Again, there is plenty to go around. Plenty of fish in the sea. A universe of total abundance.

So, if you're one of those people that hoard your belongings, worries about where money will come from or mistrusts the guidance of a supportive higher power- now is the time to change and guess what? You're in the right place. Let's keep moving forward…

To Our Final Resting Place

No, I don't mean six feet under. The final mistaken mindset we all ought to avoid is negativity and yes, this surely does sound like a lot of the above. That's because it is. You're right about that.

Negative feelings, language and action all come from the thoughts inside of your mind. That is the reason it is so important to be mindful of how you think, speak, and ultimately act. As we talked about in this very chapter, we need to be mindful of our self-talk. Is it off-putting? Do you talk poorly of yourself and your work? Are you like I used to be? Full of gossip, drama, hate and blame in the workplace?

Just some final things to think about before we shift into our next phase of this book… the seven mindsets necessary for success. Ready to read some upbeat and energizing stuff? Me too! Moving forward; rock on…

Chapter 3
How to Think Like a Successful Nurse

It's time to breathe easier now. The 'Negative Nancy' is behind us. While chapters one and two were thick, heavy and filled with dense energy which were necessary for us to sort through; the rest of this book is filled with content that is uplifting, inspiring and can help us all make changes that will impact our careers.

I find it fascinating just how intense the previous chapters have been. I could literally feel the drain as I typed the words out on the page. After reading, re-reading, editing and re-editing them; I felt tired. I speak to this energetic vibration in my previous writing and in all of my talks. You can literally feel the energy of a thought, a word and/or an action. Take pause for a moment, before we get into the light and easy content of this book, to just notice how you feel right now.

As we recently finished discussing, what we think about we certainly do bring about. If we are focused on heavy, dense and draining topics that tire us out then it's no wonder that our careers have been literally sucking the life out of us. Yet, when we move our attention to solutions, the answers to our problems, and the outcomes we'd like to experience in our careers- things get much, much easier (and more enjoyable!).

So, let's move into the content of this next chapter and let me point out right up front that these concepts are not novel ideas.

In fact, these universal laws have been around since the beginning of mankind and what's more? These truths are working, whether or not we believe in them. The laws are at work- if we are aware of them or not!

Open Your Mind

One of my favorite quotes is from a monk and teacher named Suzuki who once said, "In the beginner's mind there are many possibilities, but in the expert's mind there are few."

As we go through this chapter, some of the concepts may be new to you. Others you may have heard somewhere else before. When we receive material that we already have strong opinions around, there is a tendency to reject or accept it- based on our past experiences. Whether or not you know about these laws is actually irrelevant. What's important is that you allow yourself to open up to the information.

I encourage you to read this chapter with an open mind. This chapter actually provides the foundation for the rest of the book.

Success Thrives

In the introduction section I mentioned studying with many coaches, entrepreneurs and successful teachers. In addition to learning from and modeling the great ones, I love to read. My book shelves are lined with spiritual writings, entrepreneurial texts and inspirational guides. I have podcasts, webinars and videos galore that I often refer back to so by learning from me, you are getting access to all of these great role models and teachers (just check out the appendix for further reading and resources).

Why have I studied so much? What is with my seemingly constant need for further education? How come I continue to pay people money to help me as a nurse entrepreneur? Because these people are successful! They have what I want. They do what I'd love to do on a daily basis. They live the lifestyle that I dream of and envision myself to be living each day.

As one of my great teachers, Dr. Robert Anthony (see the appendix for his work), has said many times: don't take relationship advice from someone who can't seem to keep a companion. Avoid being counseled on money matters from a person who is broke. You get the picture. That's exactly what I did...

The great ones have written about these universal laws. Philosophers, thinkers, inventors and visionaries throughout time are quoted on these ideas. Here are just a few examples which highlight the thriving success of the universal truths:

"What this power is, I cannot say... all I know is that it exists." - Alexander Graham Bell

"A man is made by his belief. As he believes, so he is." - Bhagavad Gita

"Act enthusiastic... and you will be enthusiastic." - Andrew Carnegie

"All things whatsoever ye pray and ask for, believe that ye have received them and ye shall receive them." - The Bible

"The empires of the future are the empires of the mind." - Winston Churchill

"He is able… who thinks he is able." - Buddha

"Change the way you look at things and the things you look at change." - Wayne Dyer

Proof is in the Outcome

So you don't need to my word for it. You don't even need to listen to the great ones above. What this book is all about, what I believe of all life learning, is that you come to understand for yourself.

I always say- we can't make other people change. There is no reason to try to force people to think the way you do. It is futile for us to attempt to control another human being. I can't make you do something. I can't convince you of anything.

You've got to do the work. You're reading the book and will receive the information. You can choose to ignore it. You can decide to apply it. You can question it, looking for further knowledge and resources on such topics. In fact, that's what I would do.

I'd read the book, reflect on the material and then try out what I choose to. Then, after putting something new into practice, I'd watch my life. Am I getting the outcomes I am looking for? Do I feel better? Is my day more enjoyable? Am I finding more meaning and value from my career?

I encourage you to do the same. Go through this chapter. Think about what you read. Put into practice what you choose and see what happens. As Pamela Miles has said about Reiki Practice, "You don't have to believe in it to benefit from it. In fact, think of your first few experiences as an experiment. Observe the experience and note how you feel before and after it."

The Laws

Some say there are seven universal laws. Others state there are 12, 20 or even more. To me, it's irrelevant as to how many there actually are; we could go back and forth on this all day. What *IS* important is leading through example. I believe in teaching what one knows (and actually does). So, what I am sharing here with you below are the universal laws I have studied, reflected upon, applied and even seen work in my own life (and career).

One final 'caveat', if you will. What we'll do here is go through these universal laws and then the pages that follow will take us through practical applications. In each of the upcoming chapters, I will provide real life examples and teach actual solutions that you can choose to use with respect to your nursing career. So you will get the conceptual framework here and then put that into practice throughout the rest of this book. Sound good? OK, let's get to it.

Law of Divine Oneness

This first law speaks to connection. Everything we think, say and do has an effect on the world around us. This truth helps us to realize that we are never alone. Even in the direst of situations, when we feel isolated and as if there is no way in the world anyone can understand us, we are supported.

We can further analyze this law in relationship to energy. Since we are made of energy, as well as every single thing around us, we are all united by this energetic bond. While we certainly are physical beings, we also have some sort of 'spirit' inside of us. However you relate to your higher power, you can rest assured that this higher self is a part of you. The spirit inside of me is connected to that which is inside of you. The spirit in us all is connected to everything around and in our entire world.

As we reflect on our nursing jobs, maybe feeling at times that we have no control over our healthcare environments, we can turn to the law of divine oneness for strength. At work, have you ever felt like your efforts were in vain? Is there anything about your job that makes you feel hopeless, powerless or out of control? Have you given up on the healthcare system?

This universal law empowers us. When we realize that everything we think, say and do actually does have an effect on our experiences we can become a part of the solution. We certainly *can* impact change, one individual at a time.

Law of Vibration

We've actually already touched on aspects of this law throughout the previous chapters in this book. Remember I pointed out how the topics in chapters one and two felt very dense, very heavy and then I started out this chapter letting you know that we'd be moving on to lighter, more upbeat topics?

Well this law is all about movement. Everything in the universe moves in circular patterns and this is applicable in the physical world, because of the above (Law of Divine Oneness), we can understand that this also applies in our emotional, mental and energetic worlds as well.

This means that every thought you think, every word you say and every action you do has its own vibrational frequency attached to it. Think about it this way: what happens if you are very angry? Bring to mind a time when you were furious. Something happened at work which simply made your blood boil.

How does that feel in your body? What type of energy is associated with these feelings?

Now think about another experience- one that brought you great joy. Maybe your team accomplished a difficult task together or you received a major award at work. How does that feel in the body? A bit lighter, perhaps?

Another wonderful benefit that comes from this law is our realization that nothing is permanent. Since the law states that everything is in movement and that circular patterns exist, we can rest easy when a challenging situation comes our way. Because guess what?

If everything is in circular motion, then we can allow the difficult experience to be as it is. With the trust and acceptance that "this too shall pass", we enjoy the natural flow. This allows us to let go of attaching ourselves to anything uncomfortable since we are blessed with constant movement.

Law of Cause and Effect

This may be a law that some people struggle with. Since there are people out there who believe in luck, chance or superstitions- this may be an area that is challenging.

This truth speaks to the fact that there is no coincidence. Nothing happens by chance. Everything that we do: our thoughts, words and actions has a consequential outcome attached to it.

What's wonderful about this law is that it enables us to eliminate any type of victim role in our lives (and jobs).

This law enables us to take ownership. When we apply this truth to our lives, we become accountable for every single situation we find ourselves in. Here's a practical example for you, one that I hope you can relate to.

Think about your work place. Is there a person that you just don't mesh well with? Someone who gets under your skin. Maybe a boss, supervisor or colleague that you never seem to see eye-to-eye with?

If you have someone in mind, turn your attention to your conversations with colleagues, friends or family members. What happens when you get home from a long day of work? Let's just say this person offered you some constructive feedback. You come home and do what? Vent to your spouse, friend or neighbor.

You find yourself constantly complaining about this individual. You cannot stand their behavior. How dare they talk to you that way! Don't they know that you're trying your best? This goes on and on and you find yourself completely resenting this person and feeling as if every time you have to interact with them it may just be the last straw.

Guess what? This universal law actually puts the ownership on us. Since there is a cause and effect to every action (or inaction), we can take responsibility for the difficult relationships we find ourselves in. According to this law, we have a part in them too!

Law of Attraction

I'm sure you heard of this one before. The Law of Attraction has gotten a lot of attention thanks to the book and movie, 'The Secret'. Some folks may even have opinions regarding this law, down putting it since it has gone 'mainstream'.

However, this law, just like all of the other universal truths, is at work whether we believe in it or not (whether we agree with it or not). So, maybe we can let some of that judgment go and just open up to what this law is all about?

In the most simplest of terms, this law states that like attracts like. A lot of what we have already covered in the previous chapters of this book can be supported by this universal truth. Every thought, feeling, word and action attracts to us that which has a similar energy. We think about negating things; we get negative outcomes. We speak to others in a positive way; we experience positive relationships.

Pretty basic, huh? Let me ask you this- are you aware of this law and how it plays out in your nursing career?

Law of Relativity

As of recently, this universal law is actually one of my favorites. Last year I read a book by an author named M. J. Ryan called 'The Power of Patience'. While a lot struck me in this text, there was one concept I will never forget.

People are doing the best that they can with what they currently have (or something along those lines). This notion is synonymous with this universal law. The Law of Relativity is about how everything is, for lack of a better term, relative. No matter how bad you perceive your own situation to be, remember there is somebody out there who has it harder than you do.

This can put a lot of our nursing career drama into perspective. If we're at work, upset over our schedule, patient load or salary can we just stop a moment to think about how good we really *do* have it? We're actually *at* work. We receive a paycheck. We live with a roof over our heads. We're not the one lying in that hospital bed.

The next time you hear yourself complain (and remember-what you think or speak is reflected back to you based on the previous laws above), stop. Take a breath. Make a conscious effort to pause and ask yourself, '*Is it really that bad? Is there someone out there who has it worse than I do?*'

Kind of makes it a little bit easier to choose how to act, huh?

Law of Polarity

I recently learned this law. I started following a really great podcast by an extremely successful entrepreneur named David Neagle (see Appendix for resources). In one of his lessons, he introduced this law.

In making his point, David suggested that we think about a marker. Bring an image of a marker to mind (you know, the kind you may be using to highlight this book). What does every marker have? That's right; a tip and an end. It wouldn't be a marker if it didn't have two sides.

This universal law states that everything has an equal and exact opposite. This law is really, really cool. Since everything has an exact opposite we can use this to our advantage. When we think of something undesirable, if we are conscious and aware of our thoughts, we can immediately shift to the exact opposite.

This is really great news, because what this means is, we do not have to fall victim to our monkey mind. The more awareness we practice, the more conscious we are of our thoughts, the more empowered we become to *do* something about them. In the very moment that it happens, we can choose to shift our thoughts from a negative to its exact opposite. You got it! Every negative has a positive polarity.

Another really neat concept which David covers (and we will go into further detail on later) is how this law enables us to look for opportunity. If everything has an exact opposite, then we can look at our nursing careers in a brand new way. When there is something that you don't like about your nursing job, you can shift that focus onto what you do want to see in your role. Looking for the *exact opposite* of what you don't currently have and you will start to see your career in a very different light.

Law of Rhythm

This law is similar to the Law of Vibration, yet takes things a step further. The Law of Rhythm refers to cycles. Think about the seasons, moon cycles, or rising and falling tide. Everything comes and goes. Waxes and wanes. Things are constantly in motion. They are a part of a pattern.

More good news for us! As we learned in the Law of Vibration, we don't have to stay 'stuck' in a negative energy. We can allow ourselves to let go of negative thought or action, trusting that it is part of the natural cycle of flow. Negative comes and goes. When we choose to shift our focus, leaving the negative mindsets, we allow for natural rhythms to develop. We can learn from difficult times.

You may already recognize this in your work as a nurse. Think about an inpatient unit. What usually happens? Sometimes the unit is extremely acute. You don't seem to have enough staff and you wonder how you will ever get through it. On the other hand, other times things are (dare I say) quiet. Patient census is low and you actually have time to breathe (and eat).

So, what's the good news? Now that you are aware of this law, the next time you find yourself in a 'stressful' work situation, you can exhale and relax. You now know that a challenging time at work will also come and go.

Piecing It All Together

Well, how do you feel? Empowered? Enlightened? Excited? I surely feel that this chapter has been much more uplifting and inspiring than the previous two. I am also really eager to see how you put this all into place. (Visit the Your Next Shift Facebook Group https://www.facebook.com/groups/YourNextShift to stay connected and keep us posted.)

Take some time over the next several days to reflect on what you have read. Which law spoke to you the most? What truth surprised you? Do you disagree with any of them? How can you allow these concepts to impact your career (your life)?

We're getting ready to take these theoretical ideas and move them into actual practical experience. The next parts of this book, as I shared a bit with you earlier, will apply these notions to our real world setting (especially as it relates to our job). So, take a breather. Give yourself some room. Allow what you just read to settle in some and then come along with me as we put process into action…

Part Two

Nine Practical Applications for Your Nursing Career

We're moving into a new section of this book. I understand that for the moment, shifting into this next part of the book may feel a bit choppy and that's perfectly normal. My expectation is that this all comes together for you as we move through the next sections of the book. In the previous chapters, we've been covering things on a more conceptual level. Guess what? That was totally on purpose.

My aim was to provide you with an overarching theoretical framework first before moving into real life application. Let's revisit the purpose of this entire book: it is to give you solutions that allow you to experience more joy in your nursing practice. My goal is for you to walk away from reading this book with two things: the knowledge *AND* the skills to more greatly enjoy your nursing career.

The way I see it is that both parts of this book are entirely necessary to give you everything that you need to move forward. I'd be doing you a disservice if we jumped right into the practical applications, skipping over the universal laws that make up the mindset. I would leave out so much of the solutions you desire if I just covered the mindset and failed to apply it to any real world setting.

So, that's what we will do in the next ten chapters that follow. Please note: they may be shorter chapters than the ones prior and that is just fine. (In fact, I actually set it up that way on purpose.) I'll share an example from my own real life lessons learned and then walk you through the tool. Then, I'll ask you some reflection questions and my hope is that you take some time to do the introspection that is required.

Sure, there also may be many, many others than just the ten tips that we cover here, but, who's to say there isn't another book out there (or inside of me) that will bring more of these tools to the table? Let's start with ten and see if we can enjoy some shifts. What do you say?

I'm ready to roll my sleeves up and do the work. Are you? Let's get to it!

Chapter 4
Enjoyment Now Breeds Success Later

I am seeing the light. I am OK with where I am at right now (finally).

I've been placed on this 'project' at w-o-r-k -that while I would love to be creating my own projects- I can see that where I am is where I am meant to be. Here's what's happening...

I had a call yesterday with a nurse entrepreneur and my project coordinator who are helping me with the website move and rebranding over to www.elizabethscala.com. When we got on the line he kept asking all of these questions about my 'buckets'; who I want to work with; where do I see income coming from; what do I like to do? That got me thinking: "What does this all have to do with my website??"

Well, long story short... I finally came to the realization that I am ready to make the corporate world of nursing my 'target market'. (WOW, I can't believe I just typed that. So many emotions come with it: fear, excitement, pride, joy, doubt, readiness, professionalism, etc.) Any way... I claimed that. Really owned it. And that's what we are going to focus on with the website move and re-branding.

That said- today at work... on this new project... I am put into these groups as a silent observer. I am just supposed to sit there, take notes, and watch what I see. The groups consist of either nurse managers or bedside nurses (separate groups, asked the same questions).

WOW- The themes, information, vents, complaints, struggles, joys, challenges, etc. that I am hearing in these rooms are TOTALLY what is going to help me know how to speak to these corporate nursing markets I seek.

I am EXACTLY where I need to be right now. I am OK with my part-time role as it is serving me in my business. I know that I am meant to be a successful entrepreneur, but that there are things I am receiving and learning right now that will help me to be even HUGER (is that a word, LOL) as I get out of the gate!

Oh boy! I love this. I am ready!!!

Alicia Forest*, on our next call, we will have to re-look at the 2013 strategic plan with a really deliberate eye as to how I can position myself with my offers next year to start to 'be' that expert.

I am excited!!!!!

* Please note: I checked with my coach and others in the group and they were OK with me using their names the way that you see them here.

This was a post placed in my coaching group the winter of 2012. At that time, I was working part-time while building my business. As I shared with you in the start of this book, my business has certainly evolved over the years. I started out offering one-on-one coaching. I then moved into group program work. My website domain names (as you read above) even shifted. There are a lot of moving parts as one takes on the world of nurse entrepreneur.

Yet, there are also a lot of moving parts in the world of any nursing career. Think about your current role. I am sure there are many things you have to frequently learn to keep up with the ever-changing pace of healthcare. There are new procedures and policies that get introduced; there is innovative equipment and technology being put into place. Numerous things are shifting and to be a successful nurse you have to keep up with the changing times.

Amidst all of this change, there can be a variety of feelings. You may encounter a feeling of loss, wanting things to go back to the comfortable way that they were. You could feel resentment if the changes are felt to be placed upon you, instead of shifts that bring your decision making skills to the table. Or, you may feel a sense of impatience, excitement or urgency if you really, really want something to happen.

For me- I really, really wanted to be a nurse entrepreneur. I wanted to leave my part-time j-o-b all of the time. At times I would get so pissed off just having to get up in the morning and drive into work. I'd think to myself, *This is such a waste of time. I could be working on X, Y, and Z that will help me build and grow my business.* The post above I placed in my coaching group, which is a perfect example that reminds us to be OK with where we are right now.

I recently received an email from one of my teachers, Dr. Robert Anthony, wishing us all a happy and healthy holiday time of year. In the email, Dr. Anthony mentioned one of the reasons that many of us fail to reach our New Year's goals. He wrote about the way we set goals and how we perceive our success around whether or not we reach them. According to Dr. Anthony, this actually sets us up for failure.

Instead of judging ourselves based on whether or not we have successfully obtained a goal, Dr. Anthony encourages us to look at how far we have come. This becomes such a beautiful gift, one that can surely propel us forward.

Recognize how far you have come within your nursing career. Think back to your very first day, maybe even before that. Think back to nursing school and the tests you had to pass to become a nurse! You have accomplished so much within your nursing practice. You have achieved many goals and have come a long, long way. You know more now than you did a year ago. You know more than you did an entire career ago.

When you are OK with where you are currently at, you are able to celebrate everything about you and then exude that energy out into the world. Other people can see, feel and even experience this confident and clear individual. They will desire to be around you, wanting to work with you and engage in your presence. You will literally attract the right people, experiences and situations to you.

So, think about yourself and your current nursing career. Let's even take a real life example here. Say you are in a job that you don't really like. You want to do something different, so you've been putting your resume out all over the place. The longer it takes to find a job, the more frustrated you become. You start to doubt yourself and your ability and everything about finding a new place to work. You may even begin to dislike your current job more and more as you get irritated with the job search process.

Well, what does this do to your chances of finding new work? That's right! It kills them. Here's another real life example and while it may not be about a nurse, it certainly applies here.

My husband lost his job one fall awhile ago. He came home from work during the day, which was not usual for him because he worked in heating and air conditioning, so the majority of his day was spent driving from appointment to appointment.

Well, that day I knew something was wrong. He was home at 10 am and the van was nowhere in sight. When he came in the house all he said to me was: "I'll talk to you later." His face was red and I could tell he was really, really upset.

I gave him a moment and then went out the garage. He was unloading all of his tools and equipment from the driveway into the garage. "I lost my job today." That was that. Now, in the moment, at first I was in a state of total shock. Then, it moved into some quick worry and then something happened that was monumental.

My husband came into my home office and said to me: "What's done is done. Instead of focusing on the bad; I am looking at this as an opportunity. I wasn't really happy there and I bet I can get an even better job." And he was right.

In less than two weeks he had a better job; closer to home that provided him with a substantial raise. We were both beyond thrilled and it only gave me further validation that worry and fear don't move us forward in uncertain situations...

I've spoken and written on this point many times in the past, so I won't overdo it here. But, in brief it is important to note that we cannot change the past. We cannot control things outside of our power. Just as my husband did in the example above by choosing to approach his current career circumstances with an open mind, he realized that the energy he brought to his job hunt would definitely impact his chances at finding work (and fast).

Again, be OK with where you are at in your current nursing role. Everything happens for a reason and maybe you are in the role that you are in to learn something in particular. Maybe you are there to teach or give something to another being. There is a reason why you are working or not working where you are at in this current moment.

Be patient on the path to forward progress. Recognize the growth behind you. When you can accept where you are at now and are able to celebrate everything about it then you exude that energy out to those around you.

Self-Reflection Exercises

Where are you with respect to your career? Take an honest inventory of your job. What about your role do you enjoy?

What do you think your current situation is teaching you? What lessons can you learn from your career at this point in time?

If you are looking to make a career change, how have you been showing up in this experience? Think about the Law of Cause and Effect (chapter three). How does your thoughts, feelings, energy and actions impact your role in your job search?

Chapter 5
Clearly Plan Your Role in the Future

We always get asked the same questions at the beginning and end of the week in the coaching group I am in. The questions we receive are the following:

How did we do with our previous week commitments?

What are we focused on in the upcoming week (up to three items)?

At first, I found this process to be tedious, even annoying. I viewed it as so repetitive that I doubted writing an answer down would actually 'do' anything. To be honest, I didn't even really want to participate with the questions each week.

Then, something amazing happened. As I got to look back on what I wrote at the start of the week, I realized how many things I was able to check off that I had done. In fact, many times I am able to report that I got more accomplished than I even stated I would. I realize that it definitely serves me to do this process each Monday morning with our group as it moves me and my business forward towards my goals.

Now, this chapter may totally confuse you. It may even bother you a bit. In the last chapter, I told you to stay in the present moment as it relates to your career. While in this chapter, I am encouraging you to set your sights on the future. Why is this?

Even though it is best for us to remain calm and content in our present moments (as best we can) it serves us to look towards our future and set goals to work toward. It helps us to know where we are going. Think about it; would you ever take a trip without having a plan? The very best way to plan your future goals is to have a clear vision of what you want to have happen.

As a nurse entrepreneur, one of the things I do is I write. I am able to post articles to my own blog, while also submitting guest posts to other nurse blogger's sites. I've written about this next tip in several places. In fact, one of my dear colleagues, Beth Boynton, writes a well-known online blog called Confident Voices (see Appendix).

One time, a long while back, I wrote a guest post for her about the Law of Attraction as it pertained to nursing. That very post received more comments and feedback than any other blog post I had ever written. Beth kept emailing me over and over again, '*You got another comment on your post... Here's another response to your blog...*'

In the post that I contributed to Beth's blog, I talked about how we approach our nursing careers and our future goals. I shared that the best way for us to get what we want is to focus on it and I encouraged the readers to do just that. I warned that often we find it easier to focus on what it is that we do not want, instead of giving attention to what it is we do want.

So, I urge you to do the same. Think about your nursing career. Do you find yourself complaining about it? Have you ever vented to a colleague about something that you don't enjoy in the workplace? These are practices that keep our mindsets focused on that which we do not want and these are things (the things that we do not want) that in no way, shape or form move us forward.

If we want to move closer to our future goals, we have to shift our focus. We've got to pay attention to what it is that we do want instead of what we don't want. I actually take people through this type of exercise in many of my speeches and presentations. So let's do it in brief here together.

Think about your career. Take out a blank sheet of paper and list out everything you don't like. Write down the things you don't want to do. When you think about the negative aspects of your work, what comes to mind? Write that down. This first list is your list of 'don't wants'.

Now, take out another blank sheet of paper. Keeping your 'don't want' list in front of you, create your 'want' statements. Taking each sentence, one-by-one, reverse them to the exact opposite. You may find it helpful to say something like this to yourself: *'If I don't want X, then what I do want is Y.'*

We're doing this here together for practice, but you can do this as you go about your work day. As you practice nursing, observe yourself. Where do you find yourself feeling negative, stuck or as if you don't like what is happening around you? How can you shift your focus in that moment to what it is you do want to have happen?

As you use this tool, you will find that your decisions come easier. Let's just say you are a nurse entrepreneur or that you would like to be one. When you come to work for yourself and own your own company, you will be faced with tons of options. You may have to make decisions on a daily basis! How will you decide what is the best thing to do and what will help you know which way to go? When you keep your future vision in mind, the one that pertains to your desires, it will be easier to make difficult choices.

Even if you have no desire to travel the nurse entrepreneur path, you may be faced with career alternatives in nursing. Will you go back to school? Should you get a specialty certification? Does it make sense to take that extra training or go through the advanced course? Keeping your future vision close to heart, the one that deals with your wants out of life, you will be able to make the best decision.

I've often shared the story of my relationship with affirmations. For quite a while, I didn't believe in them. I didn't think that they worked. Then, I came across a spiritual teacher who explained that we are actually using affirmations all day long. Our entire life experience is the affirmations of our mind in the physical realm. What we see in our nursing careers is the product of our thoughts, the outcome of our affirmations.

If you find yourself in a nursing job that you don't fully enjoy, start to observe your thought processes. What are you focused on? Do you spend the majority of time in thought about what it is you do not want? Is there room for a shift to staying mindful of what it is that you do want? Can you allow this shift to move you forward to the nursing career of your dreams?

Self Reflection Exercises

Take time to go through the exercises above that pertain to your "don't want" and "do want" lists.

Write down a very clear vision of what you want your future nursing career to look and feel like.

What one step can you take today to move you closer to your goals tomorrow?

Chapter 6
Trust in the Process of Patient Flow

Just thought I'd share where I am at since I won't be able to make today's call. I am feeling no-movement. I don't have much income coming in. I don't do much 'work' since I am not creating any programs, products or trying to get coaching clients. I've been sending out emails and follow-up emails, offering my speaking services, with not much response. How can I leave a job if I don't have income coming in from my business? Yes, that age-old question again.

I continue to trust that I am on the right path and even more than that, if I am not, I am supported anyway. I do believe this is a good universe, a kind world. I do believe that no matter what happens, I will always have what I need. I am sure I am OK. It is just scary. The unknown. The desire to want something so badly; to know where I want to go, but not see much progress forward.

When I look back, yes the progress is there. It's a matter of patience, expectations, wanting control. That is still where I have room to grow. I want what I think I want and I want it now. Letting go of control and knowing 'how' these things will happen and turn out is tricky. Being a recovering 'control-aholic' it's hard to know what's what.

My final worry is this: what if the years of trying, working at it, sometimes forcing (?) this entrepreneurial me is 'all wrong'. The universe supports the path that I am most meant to help and serve on. What if I have this plan of being this 'speaker/writer' for nurses and that is all wrong? Then, it's no wonder that I haven't seen things pan out financially. It's no wonder people don't get back to me. Sure, this could just be the smaller me sabotaging myself. So, I keep pressing forward. But, when is the press forward the wrong press?

You know what I would love? A sign. I hear about all of these people getting 'clear signs' and 'messages'. They know they are on the right track. They know they are living their purpose. Many days I do my meditation and practices, I ask the universe for a sign. I say I am ready to be guided. I am vulnerable. I am open. I am ready for support. Show me the way.

I just haven't seen that sign. Or maybe I missed it!

I am actually feeling positive. I continue with all of my self-care practices and feel really, really good about my life. The scary stuff is the 'how will' it happen and 'when'. The signs are desired and I'd love to be completely self-employed and that's just that.

In fact, the desire to be totally self-employed is what's gotten me out of the fear of calling people, that fear of rejection. I don't care anymore. I continue to follow up because I am going for what I want. Now, if I am going for what I want, can't the universe meet me half-way and give me a bit of help out?

Yup; that was me. That post above was the very words I shared with my coaching group some years back. And as I re-read it to put into this book I thought to myself, 'Wow. Sometimes I still feel this way.' Want to know what happened next?

My very next thought was this: 'At least these thoughts and feelings come less frequently. At least I know what to do with them now. At least I have practices to help me through…'

This next tool for you is simple. One of my dear colleagues (and I can't believe I cannot remember which one it was; I always like to give credit where it is due) said to me once on one of my radio show episodes: what is simple isn't always easy. Profound words of wisdom that are so true. What we say is 'simple' doesn't always turn out to be 'easy' to do or practice. The tool I am about to give you is simple in that it is understandable enough in essence, so here it is.

You need to continue to trust when the going gets tough. Let go of 'how' it is going to happen for you and believe in the process. Leave behind any need to know 'when' you will get the outcomes you desire; know that it is coming if not already there.

One of the intentional affirmation statements I use quite often is this: 'I choose to let go of any attachment to expectation or outcome. I choose to let go of the need to control and trust in the flow of life.' Sometimes easier said than done, right? As I said from the advice shared with me by many wise colleagues: it may sound simple, but won't always be easy.

Being a nurse entrepreneur, there is a lot of trust and letting go that happens. In fact, I have note cards hanging up all around my office to remind me of this very notion. Part of being in business for yourself means that you have the autonomy and freedom to flex your creativity muscles. When you get innovative and start to build programs, products and services to offer you want things to produce results. Sometimes, it takes a bit of time, growth, and patience for things to take hold and produce the traction that you are looking for.

Think about your nursing career. Is there something you would like to see differently? Is there a job change you are hoping to make? Let me ask you a harder, more personal question. Are you attempting to force the outcome you think should happen?

Yes, we need to have goals. As we covered in chapter five, it makes sense for us to plan our future and be a proactive component of our career path. However, when we are butting our heads up against the wall, time and time again, is it possible that the universe is trying to send us a message? Is there a place that we need to tune in and listen up? I'll give you another example from my experience...

In my part-time job, I was getting ready to lead my own research study. Well, when I say 'ready' I mean three years in the making ready. Sure, research takes a lot of time and there are many moving parts, but this was getting to be just nuts.

Every single brick wall that could have reared its ugly head did. I had to go in front of an extra review board (multiple times) and defend my work. I had to go to physician meetings and practically beg for their support. I had to register the study as a clinical trial, obtain a biosafety number, and jump through more hoops than any other study I had been involved with before.

Then, there was my Primary Investigator (or should I say investigators, plural?). The first one left my organization; the second one left the state. I had to put in multiple changes to my research protocol and there were so many technicality holdups. Personnel kept changing and people kept coming and going from the study team. After awhile, I started to realize… maybe this wasn't meant to be.

I started to talk to my final and current PI about how I was feeling. She wanted me to push forward, saying that it wasn't the research idea that was getting denied. It was just all of these technical issues that were really silly and insignificant. And sure, on the one hand that was true, but on the other hand, because I believe in the concepts of universal laws and letting go of forced control, I saw it another way.

After much conversation, I must have finally made my case, because she let me withdraw the study. I had never formally 'quit' something before. Even as a kid when I was cut from a basketball team, my mother and I fought the coach for my spot back on the roster. So, I didn't know how it would feel. Would I be ashamed? Am I a failure? Is this the wrong decision?

I received my confirmation and it didn't come from the reactions (or lack thereof) from others. It didn't come in some outlandish sign. In fact, it came from within. I felt 'right' with this choice and space has been freed up to focus on other aspects of my career…

Sometimes, we may be looking for some extravagant sign from the universe, but we never get it. Often, the answer lies within. When we become quiet and tune into our own feelings, we can receive profound answers.

This is true with our nursing career. Whether or not you are looking to make a change, the answers lie within. If the going gets tough and you're unsure which way to go, let go of any attachment to 'how' things will happen or change. Remember, practicing patience is key.

Self Reflection Exercises

What does the term 'attachment' mean to you? Is there anywhere in your nursing career that you have become attached to an outcome or expectation?

Is there anything you are trying to change with respect to your nursing practice and if so, what may you be forcing? Is there anything that needs a lighter grip?

How can you open up to subtle signs of support? In what ways can you go with the flow of life?

Chapter 7
Shift Your Focus

My post today is short and sweet. I received a comment on my blog. Here is what it said…

"Your articles have sparked an interest in nursing that I had lost a long time ago. You have actually given me Hope."

This is what Nursing from Within™ is all about. I feel so full of gratitude that my writing is helping another nurse reconnect with the joy.

Last year I went to my coach's live event. During this event, she has us touch base with the 'why' behind our business. She has us do some introspective exercises to tap into the reasons beneath why we do what we do as entrepreneurs.

Now I've done this exercise many, many times. In fact, I have done it not only with my business coach but with other spiritual guides and teachers as well. So, I'm used to it and I've always thought I've known the real reasons *why* I want to be a nurse entrepreneur.

Well, this year something shifted. Something really special happened. You might even call it an 'a-ha' moment.

I am very aware of the reasons why I want to work for myself. I want freedom and autonomy. I want a flexible schedule and the convenience of working from home. You know- those sorts of things everyone secretly wants from their j-o-b.

Of course, I also want to work for myself for larger reasons. As I shared in the introduction of this book, I've always missed working in direct patient care. One of my beliefs is that by working with the clinical nurses who interact with patients each day that I am somehow indirectly affecting the care that they receive. On a more global level, a major intention of my business is to make a huge impact on healthcare and the nursing profession overall.

But, you know what came out last year that was very different than any other thing I have said, felt or written down before? I wrote something on my paper that struck a chord deep inside. I wrote something down so meaningful that I actually raised my hand to share it with the group (something I seldom do in large rooms like that).

I realized that my intention of becoming a nurse entrepreneur is to be of service to others. That's what the tool in this chapter is all about. It's about shifting your focus from how you can help yourself and your career to how you can serve others so that it meaningfully impacts your nursing practice.

Guess what? You can do this in any and every role out there in the nursing profession. Think about this example. Say you are looking to get a new job. You have to go on an interview usually, right? Well when you're in that 'hot seat' instead of answering the questions in the usual way (the way that highlights all of the reasons that you're perfect for the job) think about answering the questions in a way that shows how you can serve that manager, that unit, the staff team or the organization that you will be joining.

In the business world we call this the 'what's in it for them' thinking. You may even see entrepreneurs out there use the acronym WIFT. We want to shift our focus from serving us and our wants and needs to how we can serve others and I bet for you as a nurse, this one will be an easier tool to add to your kit since naturally we are used to helping other people.

However, I want you to take this a step further. It's more than taking care of others. It's about figuring out the problems they have and how you can offer your unique solution to them. As a nurse in a clinical role, how can you solve the issues of the workplace that will set you apart as an employee? As a budding, part-time or fully successful nurse entrepreneur, how can you ease the pain of your target market?

When you shift your focus to how you can serve another (or a group of others), it becomes so much easier for you to enjoy career success (and sustain it).

Let me give you an extra tip to take this technique to the advanced level. When you are highlighting the answers to the people whose challenges you are solving (remember, WIFT) you want to be sure to focus on the benefits instead of the features. You may be thinking, '*Huh?*' That's perfectly normal; let me explain.

Say I am offering a digital course. I have created it all virtually and because of that it comes with things like 4 thirty minute webinars, 2 Q&A conference calls and a secret Facebook group. Well, those things I just listed, those are the features. So, what are the benefits? The benefits are the things that the participants actually get from the webinars, conference calls and Facebook group. You might think of it as a benefit comes from the features of the offer.

Benefits can be things like the support of a like-minded group. They might have someone to listen to your cluttered mind and help you come to clear conclusions. A benefit from a product like the above could very well be (depending on the content) enjoying a more meaningful career that provides you with a more lucrative income. See what I mean? Benefits tap more into feelings and emotions while features just state what the offered solution looks like (what it's made up of).

So again, let's relate this to your nursing career. Let's say you are trying to solve a problem of a colleague, staff member or boss. While it's great to point out to them your nifty solution (the feature), it may serve you to also highlight how it will benefit them.

How will they feel? What will they gain? In what way does your help solve their problem?

When I came to the realization that one of my big 'whys' behind my business was serving the nursing profession and the nurses that practice it, things got a whole lot easier. This awareness makes it easy to show up each day to the 'office' with surefire enthusiasm. I am less intimidated by putting myself out there, offering my services. It has become seemingly effortless to create products that offer solutions to the problems at hand. And the best part? It's so much more fun!

Self-Reflection Exercises

In your current nursing job, how do you view your role of service? Do you go to work to collect the salary? Are you there to solve problems and offer solutions? If so, how?

Think of your 'target market' (those people you serve each day). What problems are they challenged with? What unique solutions can you offer your target market and how will these solutions benefit them?

What does it mean to you to shift your focus to serving others through your career?

Chapter 8
Keep Getting Their Attention

Here's a question. I put out the survey to the list and got 60 responses. About 5 or so gave me their contact information to follow up and learn more on how I can help them with nurse's week. I emailed them all Monday. So far I have heard back from no one.

When is it too soon to re-email? Is Friday OK? Most people gave their phone numbers too. When is too soon to call? Next Tuesday or Thursday OK?

I have a plan that I use for reaching out to nurse associations: email 1 one week, 2 a week a few days (about ten) later, then call a week and then some more days out from that (again, about ten).

I don't know what the proper timing is on touching base. I am just doing what I do and wonder... too spaced out? Too soon? Good balance? How much and how often should I follow up?

Again, another real post from me to my coach and my coaching group. The issue here: the art of follow up. How often is too often? When does it start to feel like stalking? What is a good rule of thumb when figuring out how much to space out a second email, phone call or other form of contact?

Well that's what this chapter is all about. The tip for you here is to be consistent and persistent in your follow up. This will come as absolutely no surprise to you, but I'll say it anyway. People are busy.

Think about the digital age we live in. How many emails do you get on a daily basis? In fact, check your inbox right now. How many emails are in it? I know some people that get over a thousand emails a day. A day! I hope I never ever get that popular that I am receiving that many emails per day (LOL).

Guess what else? Not everyone checks their email on a daily basis. People don't all use their voicemail boxes that often. Another thing I've learned being a nurse entrepreneur is that we not only have to be consistent and persistent in our follow up, but we have to approach it from multiple avenues. That's why I now email, call and use snail mail to get the word out about my work.

As a nurse entrepreneur, we have many options as to how we spread the message about our products and services. There are lots of channels of communication. Some folks like to focus on social media. Others use email marketing or blogs. You can even break it down further as to how you deliver your media. Do you write? Does podcasting or audio mp3s work best for you? How about video, streaming live or using an online hangout system?

I'll say it again. People are mad busy. They are over inundated with information. You have to 'touch' people many times (and in multiple formats) to even get them to know that you exist. Being persistent with your follow up isn't overdoing it; they may not even get all of the messages that you send. If you got one thousand emails per day, I'd bet some of them would wind up never being read either.

The other thing I've mentioned, but not really focused on heavily yet is one of the key words above: consistent. The 'consistency' piece is what is going to do two things for you. One, it's going to set you apart from all of the others out there who are also trying to follow up with the same person that you are. Two, your consistency is going to show that you are serious and professional. You mean business.

'*OK,*' some of you reading might be thinking, '*Well, this tip sounds like it is extremely important for a nurse entrepreneur. But, what about me? I have no interest in owning my own business. How does this chapter's tool apply to me and my nursing career?*'

Great question. Well being that you are a nurse, in a job, with an employer- you too are going to have to follow these same rules of follow through. If you are reading this book and looking to find out some ways to get a new job that you enjoy more than your old job, well guess what? You got it. You're going to have to follow up with folks who you reach out to about a possible job change.

Let me share a resource with you that will help make your job search that much easier. It's called social media. Now, don't freak out on me. I, too, went onto social media kicking and screaming. And while it's not one of my favorite things to do as it relates to my business, social media is actually very useful and let's face it, it's not going away.

One of the best places you can be on if you are looking for a job as a nurse is LinkedIn. This social media platform is much more professional than the others. There are groups on almost every topic you can imagine that you can join. Once you get involved with a group, you want to be consistent with your participation in the discussions. You can use these groups to position yourself as an expert, answering questions and sharing solutions with group members like you.

Another thing that LinkedIn is great (and known) for is the connections. You can build your network of nurses and who knows? One day another nurse may be able to refer you for that dream job you have your eye on. LinkedIn is so much more than just about finding a job. It's about creating lasting connections that you can continue to follow up with and provide value to. All of the above pertains to those interested in nurse entrepreneurship as well and a great resource can be found in the Appendix for using LinkedIn in the best possible way.

Another caveat I will share with you here as it relates to the persistent and consistent follow up tool is this: stay organized. Especially if you are going to be using this follow up tactic as a means to growing your referral network and your product and service offer base. You want to be sure that you have a system in place that helps you keep things in a very structured and ordered way.

The worst thing to do is to start with all of this follow up and then fall off of the map because you forgot to do it. Remember, I said that consistent follow up shows professionalism? What will people think if you touch base with them one month and then don't show back up again for another six to eight months? They may start to speculate just how serious you are about your nursing career.

Finally, remember I said that it is helpful for the nurse entrepreneur to show up in multiple channels (written, audio, video, etc.)? This also pertains to the nurse who isn't necessarily looking to own her/his own business but wants to enjoy a thriving career.

Let's say, for example, you are an oncology nurse with a focus in hematological malignancy. Well, that's pretty specialized, right? Say you're working on a clinical unit; you're very satisfied and have no desire to change jobs any time soon. But, you are looking to "level-up" your career and add more value to your role. Well, what can you do?

Someone with this level of specialized knowledge may want to impact the nursing profession and the healthcare system as a whole. You might get online, set up a blog space and start posting informative and resourceful content for your patient population.   In this way, you are adding value to your own nursing career while serving your patients and their families (and on a much global scale because an internet blog can reach far beyond your local community). You feel inspired and have breathed new energy into your professional role *AND* you're getting to help others learn more about their diagnosis and disease process. It's a win-win.

There are so many ways that a nurse can be creative. Building a strong network of connections can help boost your career on many levels. Keeping and staying in touch just adds value to these special and important relationships.

Self-Reflection Exercises

What is your professional network like? Does it consist of more than just the nurses you work with on a daily basis? Take some time to list out your nursing relationships (all of them).

How can you grow your professional network? What is one way you would like to get you, your profession and your brand out there?

In what way will you stay in touch with people? Will you use social media to share content with a specific population? Will you join an online discussion forum or group? How can you up-level your career and the profession of nursing as a whole?

Chapter 9
Feel and Do: Knowledge is Power

*Holy Cow! Total celebration: these money sheets, set points, etc.
work. Last year, my money set point (what I made the most over my highest 5
paying month's average) was $862/month. This year (so far, we still have
time!), my money set point was $1675/month. Almost double.*

*So in looking out to next year, I could double the $1675. OR (my
big money goal is to increase my income by 5x), so I could go for a reach and
multiple by 5. Reading what it says on the worksheet ("set your new money set
point just outside of your comfort level").... I am going to go for a goal next
year that does that.*

*I KNOW I can double- we saw that from the above. And 5x is my
stretch...*

*So, I will make my new money set point for next year in between the
two at $6350/month. Boy that would totally work and be plenty for me to
leave my 'j-o-b' job. Let's do this!*

*Oh and PS- what's fascinating is this worksheet actually lines up
nicely with the calculation of your baseline cash flow one. On that I had
$3000/month (where I am at now at my job) as my 'break even' number. My
'peace of mind' number- I thought I would go ahead and double that to make
it easy... well, that works out to be (duh) $6,000.00/month. Which...
reverting back to the above... that new money set point of $6350/month fits
me perfectly.*

This clarity, reason and seeing it in actual black-and-white helps so much. AND will help me reach my goals. AND will help me trust in the universal support of an abundant universe! Yay!!! I am thrilled and feeling so blessed. Thanks for all of your support! Hold me to this number now guys…

Wow. The transparency. This is another actual post from me to my coaching group one year on the 'numbers'. A touchy subject for many; a tricky topic to master. While this chapter's tip is not entirely about money, it can be used in relationship to it. This might just be one of the most important tips in this part of the book so please pay attention. You ready for it? Here it is:

Fight the fear and know your numbers. Be aware of your numbers (in whatever sense that means: money, market reach, email list size, website visits, etc.) as this will empower you. Knowing where you are currently at helps you do two things. First, it can help you make the best decisions when moving forwards with a choice. Second, knowing your numbers can assist you in making changes when things need to be done differently.

Another part of this chapter's tip comes from a book by Susan Jeffers entitled 'Feel the Fear and Do It Anyway'. I actually had another experience happen similar to, yet not exactly in the same vain as the above post… which I will share as well with you.

Last winter we had a lot of 'stuff' happen. We got a security system installed in our home. We moved a ton of furniture from my parents' house in NY here to Maryland. We had the holidays, some unexpected bills and some other things come up like my husband coming onto my health insurance policy. Needless to say, my money gremlins were creeping in and I was feeling some worry over if we had enough to cover the expenses.

As I was walking up the driveway with my dog, I thought to myself: 'This is crazy. I am worried about this for no reason. I don't even know when the one bill is going through. Let me just call up the security people and ask.' Needless to say, the worry was all in vain.

A very nice and helpful woman answered the phone. She and I talked and we realized that the payment would not go through until well after I had some more money in my bank account. All was well and I hung up feeling relieved, empowered and much more content with life again.

What does the above teach us? Well, as Susan Jeffers points out, it is best to feel the fear as that is what will help us move forward into action. I could have continued to avoid how I was feeling and put off the unknowing. However, I decided to take simple action and make one phone call that liberated me for the rest of my day.

When we don't know what we don't know (or do know) it can paralyze us. That's because we are afraid of the unknown. We are afraid of change and it can keep us stuck. Procrastination actually is an action. It's an action we choose when we are afraid of moving forward towards a change.

Being a nurse entrepreneur there are lots of numbers to know. How much money is coming in and how much is going out? How many people are signed up for a free call? How many people viewed a website page? How many subscribers do I have on an email list? The numbers might go on and on… and on.

As I said before, the good thing about knowing your numbers is that it can help you make smart decisions. If you see that something worked in the past, why change it? Repurpose what worked and make your life easier. On the other hand, if you find something flopped that's actually good news because you know (by knowing your numbers) what you could do differently and where/how so that you can turn it into success next time. Or, it can tell you to let that idea go and move onto something different.

Being that the above is speaking to the nurse entrepreneur and the things they will need to know in business, what about the clinical nurse? Well to be honest with you, it's the same exact thing.

Even if you aren't a business owner, you still have to manage your money. Using money as the example because money is typically the thing that most people struggle with, you have to know how much is coming in versus going out. You have to balance your checkbook (who has one anymore? I do!); manage your bills; and plan for the future. Having the awareness of what is happening with your numbers can help you take the best, most informed action steps forward.

Another reason knowing your numbers (as a nurse entrepreneur or not) is useful is because it can give you great insight into where you may or may not need help. And we can all use support systems, whether or not we are in business for ourselves.

Just as my first share in this chapter depicted, knowing our numbers can also give a great sense of satisfaction. Had I not taken the time to go through the money worksheets provided to me by my coach, I may not have ever realized that I actually *did* double my income that year. And the year before that and before that!

This is so critical since we all have a tendency to be harder on ourselves than we need to be. When we are in the moment and living in the current day-to-day expenses, we may not have an awareness that our income actually has increased. But when we take the time to actually look things over it provides clarity for success. It shows us another accomplishment that we can celebrate. It gives us a really great reason to feel good about ourselves and the work that we do.

These exercises can be really good for the clinical nurse who also has a part-time hobby that provides him/her with income. Maybe you write a blog and receive money for sponsored posts. Or maybe you are an affiliate to another nurse's product. Whatever the case may be, make sure that you are watching your numbers in totality. You might just be surprised by where the income is coming from and guess what? Those surprises can help you make educated (and lucrative) decisions going forward.

Knowledge certainly is power and having this information can move us forward towards even bigger and better goals. It is the unknown that keeps us afraid and in the dark. Shining light on your numbers truly will set you free.

Self-Reflection Exercises

What numbers frighten you? What numbers excite you? Take some time to reflect on the two and make a list of both.

How can you 'know your numbers'? Is there a way you can start to track things so that you can empower your knowledge? What type of practice, support or guidance will you need?

Be honest with yourself. How do you feel about money? What is your relationship with money like? What stories do you have about money? Take some time reflecting on the money mindset you live with

Chapter 10
Celebrate the Small Stuff...
And the Middle, Big and In-Between!

I just want to thank this group from the bottom of my heart. I have seen such wonderful strides in my work and growth in my being. I am celebrating so much these days, it's hard to keep up with what I've shared with you and what I have missed!

I got a call yesterday from a person I know in Maryland, through Facebook. She has been following my work and my posts and knows I am passionate and driven. She was asked to speak at a nurse retreat in NJ, but felt I would be a better fit for the job. She asked if it was OK if she told the woman in NJ about me, referring me and my information to her. Last night she forwarded it along!

The client who came on Monday for Reiki absolutely loved it and called Tuesday to give me a 'status report' on how well he had slept. He said he would be coming back for more! (And telling his friends, family, and neighbors!)

The gym I hung a flier up at will be having an anniversary bash in the fall and wants me to come do the Reiki for their clients there.

Celebrating my Nurse's Week paid speaking event, my keynote speech in the fall, and more presentations to follow!

Celebrating my recent interactions with my email list as they are opening, clicking and following through with my Art of Nursing survey.

Celebrating how creative I was this morning as I created a special report and video for this week's email inviting them to participate in the Art of Nursing program.

I am seeing it all over social media as more and more people share the word about the Art of Nursing virtual conference. I am also celebrating the six taped interviews we already did- they were freaking amazing!!!

I am continuing as I been doing and living life full of fun, gratitude and joy. This is going so well these days!

While this tip is short and sweet, for many of us (raising my hand, here) it can be quite challenging. The tool for this chapter is this: celebrate the successes. The more you can focus on the joy, the more of it you will receive.

How come this is so hard for us? Well as nurses we are used to working hard and what happens after the hard work is over? You guessed it! There's more of it right behind that, which we just completed.

It seems as if we are always on-the-go. As a nurse entrepreneur, one product launch ends and there is another program waiting to be released out into the world right behind it. We're constantly on social media networking, collaborating and promoting our work. The blog posts never stop. The newsletter needs to be written. The radio show guests need to be briefed on what happens when they are 'live' on the air.

Working in business for one's self can seem like an around-the-clock job and it can certainly become one, if we're not careful. I fell into this trap myself actually, back in the start of my business. I remember my husband coming into my office one weekend and saying to me, '*When are you going to stop working? I thought the point of you going into business for yourself was so that you didn't have to work as much as when you did at the hospital?*'

He was right. One year I was a complete workhorse. I successfully launched my first tele-summit in the spring of one year. What happened when it was over? That's right; I took right up to planning the next one. I didn't even exhale long enough to actually enjoy the success that my first summit provided me.

In fact, moving at this fast of a pace could be the very reason we judge ourselves so harshly. It could be behind why we are always questioning, doubting and criticizing our own success. We don't come up long enough for air to even feel the benefits of all of our hard work!

Yes, sometimes what we put out there into the world isn't going to be well received. Everything we launch may not take off with 100% success. So, then there is another twist added to this chapter's tip: in every single situation there really is a 'win'.

I talked about this a bit in Chapter Eight of '*Nursing from Within*' where I wrote about my uncle's death. While the entire situation was a tragedy and to this day we all miss Billy, there is something to be taken from every single experience. We can learn, grow, heal or change from every life lesson.

It may be hard to do (and even see) at first, but there is a celebration to be experienced in every single thing that we do. I have a real life example of this that even I am shocked by as I re-read the vignette I am about to share with you...

Well, I know what you are going to say Alicia Forest. Take a breath and let everything sink in before I start to pick it apart. And to some extent, I am- I will. I am going away this weekend to Cape May with no computer what-so-ever and will totally unplug. Rest, relax, and commend myself for a job well-done.

But then... there is more (as there always is with me and my long-winded self, monkey minded craziness).

So, here are the pros and cons of the series as I am seriously questioning what to do with myself and this going forward:

Pros:
200+ signed up (my goal was 300)
made $1000+ (my goal was $2000)
hosted really awesome calls with live callers on each line
had several paid sponsors
was able to post on 6+ nursing blogs about it
during the entire months leading up to the series got a lot of new email subscribers
the private Facebook (FB) group has over 200 people in it now
uplifting chatter on the FB group and in the emails
I love being the hostess
I love doing my own webinar, of course

Cons:
the speakers were exhausting, not one of them knew what was going on or what to do and all had some issue with technology
technology issues
emails from participants who didn't read directions
speakers who did not share/post/participate
speakers whose presentations were not up-to-par
the amount of effort I put in and the return in dollars and signups
the reach that was just not getting there this time
the exhaustion from marketing
my own feeling of 'is it time to give this up? are people sick of me and my event?'

I guess that is all I can think of for now, but I am just feeling like this is so much work for little return. The saddest part of that is I enjoy the event, I love doing it, I love hosting, and I love putting it on for participants who take part in it. I just get so tired from it all and really don't get paid for anything.

I want to do a paid event next year but worry my numbers are not large enough to make any real impact.

So going forward with these, these are things I am considering (solutions):

doing a paid event (there may be less people, but then I would be paid for the energy I put out there)

offering speaker affiliate (it may attract them to promote the program more)

getting that hospital sector packet to go through (we created it, but it was only 3 weeks away when it was done and I was showing it to people... if I started that NOW for an event in May 2014 I am more likely to get it on board)

doing a shorter event with more sessions per day and at a time (like a real, in-person conference runs)

doing it during Nurses Week and going back to just for nurses

creating a specific topic for next time and leaving off the RC title (maybe people see the RC and think 'been there done that')

That's all I can think of (For now...)

Want to hear something pretty amazing? Remember I said I was shocked when I re-read the above post myself. Why did reviewing that vignette almost have me fall out of my chair? Because of everything we've been discussing so far in this book...

I was present to my experience, being in the moment and observing what I could learn from the situation at hand. I started to list out the pros and cons and then offer some solutions that I might be able to do in the future. I was much more clear (in terms of the solutions) of how a future program would look and feel. I learned from the previous tele-summits I offered several times over before. And guess what?

What you read above was the exact evolution of my Virtual Conference I put on annually during Nurse's Week. That very next year I launched the inaugural Art of Nursing program and experienced more success than I could have ever imagined. So, after reading the above, I thought to myself (again) *'Geez... these tips I am sharing with my readers really* **DO** *work.'*

OK, I feel as though I have neglected our other group of readers for some time now. I know the above is very much about being a nurse entrepreneur, so let's touch base with how this tip can be applied to a nurse who is an employee at some type of organization.

If I were a betting gal, I would wager that at this point you're already envisioning some ways that this tip might work for you in the clinical setting. However, I have one example to bring to the table of many that can highlight how you too can apply this tool in your career (wherever that may be).

What happens on typical nursing units? We have some sort of shared governance system, right? Most institutions these days have some type of professional model that includes a committee or council structure. Groups of nurses gather together at the organizational, departmental, and unit level to solve the challenges that are faced.

It has been my experience that these groups work on solving problems. It has also been my experience that these groups work in this way: from one problem to the next to the next and the next. There is little time to catch our breath and evaluate if what we worked on actually had an impact.

We've got to give ourselves a break from this type of continuous problem solving behavior. Let the dust settle before working on a new project. Take a break. Do as I shared in the example above and review the pros/cons of what was done. Evaluate if your solution worked and most importantly, as we learned about in Chapter Five, envision how you would like to move forward in the most successful way. Make sure your choices are based on what you do want to see happen and experience in the future.

So to recap, for all of us. There is something to be gleaned from every single life experience. Even those that appear at the time to be unsuccessful, what can you learn? How can you grow? In those situations that you did achieve in- make sure to actually exhale and allow yourself to feel the benefits of your hard work. Celebrate all of your successes.

Self-Reflection Exercises

What project have you recently completed? Have you graduated with a degree, received a specialty certification or been honored with some award at work? Were you able to celebrate your success?

If you don't celebrate your successes, why is that? What is one thing you can start to do to begin to shift that?

Make a list of some of the ways you can celebrate an achievement. Many of us aren't even sure how we would celebrate, so take some time here to create a list of how you would like to bask in the glory of your job well done

.

Chapter 11
Ask for Help Whether You're Aware of It or Not

I am on an airplane to Boston, MA. As I sit back and open up my backpack to work on the pre-event materials, I realize I am unsure of where I am going and why. I know I am on my way to a live event with a business coach. I know I am going because I have started up a business of my own. I just don't remember signing up or what this thing was all about.

It's fall and I do remember that this past spring I was on LinkedIn, just poking around and reading some discussion group postings. I found something that caught my attention. It was a promotion for a webinar that was going to teach us how to make six figures in less than part-time hours. Who wouldn't want to do that?

So... I signed up. I attended the webinar. I took all of the notes I could and then I signed up for the live event in New England for the fall of that year. I don't know what it was; I just felt drawn to the speaker. She had a wonderful energy and kept talking about how she puts her priorities first, even before her business. That's why I wanted to become a nurse entrepreneur. I wanted to live my life and enjoy myself around my work. Not the other way around.

As I am sitting here on the plane, I cannot even remember what the speaker of that webinar looked like. Who was this coach I was going to learn from? What was this three day event going to be all about? I started to realize that I couldn't remember why I was going and I had no clue what would happen when I got there.

Well, one of the funniest things did happen when I arrived. That very first day of the workshop I was sitting next to my roommate. The business coach at the front of the room was talking about list building and how to get our businesses out there. I was so confused. I turned to the woman sitting next to me and whispered, 'What list is she talking about?'

Boy did I need help! I didn't even know what I didn't even know. And guess what? That is the scariest place to be.

I tell this story all the time when I give a talk on becoming a nurse entrepreneur. It's funny that it all happened that way and I do realize that the above makes me sound a little silly. However, I use this example to teach us a very important lesson that we will cover in this chapter: we need to ask for support.

We need to ask for help all of the time. Even when we don't have a clear idea of what we need assistance with, even if we aren't 100% sure of our question- ask for help. Simply having the mindset that having guidance along the way really can help you move forward will make your journey that much easier. You don't have to do this alone.

One of my posts in my coaching group shows this exact principle:

This is what I need help/support with. I keep staying grounded in my affirmative statements, setting my intention for this event. I keep 'doing' the do parts of the work and also 'being' in the faith that I am a success. I continue to open up to insights, intuition, people and opportunities. Whatever comes my way and helps this thrive, I am open to.

I don't have a particular question, but just a desire for support. Thank you.

Sure, when you ask with a sense of clarity things will be delivered much faster to you. Yet in this case, I am not really talking about asking for specific things. What I am writing to here is the support that is all around you all of the time.

There are dear friends and family members that can listen to your hardships. There are business coaches and experts that can show you the systems. There are friends and peers that can understand with a sympathetic ear. The reason I am making the case for the difference in asking for help for specific items versus knowing that we are supported all of the time is because as nurses we typically do a pretty poor job in this respect.

How many times has a colleague come up to you during a shift and asked you if you needed help? What is our typical response? 'Nah, I'm fine.'

Even if we are drowning, even if nothing is going our way- we act as if we have everything under control. Sure, we are quick to jump in and offer help to another person. Yet when it comes to asking for and receiving support from another person it is a bit harder for us to do.

Now, this book isn't about figuring out the reasons why and it very well may be work that you can do on your own introspective time. Yet, I encourage you to take the tip in this chapter very seriously. Asking for help, even if you're unsure what that looks like, is something that we all need to do.

As a nurse entrepreneur, there is no way I can do it all. There just aren't enough hours in the day. I have social media to tend to, emails to send out, calls to make and clients to prepare for. I have blogs to write, radio show guests to prep and my own education and skill building so that I can stay up-to-date on the times. Networking, marketing, teaching, writing, and speaking… I've got to do it all. Right?

Wrong. I can hire help. Delegating some of the tasks out clears up my time to work on things that I enjoy. Building a team of support around me helps me get more done. And, of course, throughout this book I have been referring to my own coach and the group that I am in. I also need to get support for other things that come up.

For example, when I want to throw in the towel and have had enough or when I don't know how to approach a specific problem, or maybe just asking for help about some new technology that has come out. Having a business coach and a group going through similar things that I am has made a world of difference.

Let me just put in a plug for all of those business coaches out there. Nurses, we are not entrepreneurs at heart. Unless you were in business for yourself before your nursing degree, there is a pretty good chance that you haven't learned a thing about starting and successfully running your own company. You went to nursing school like me, didn't you? They didn't teach us a thing about entrepreneurial start-ups, right! Business coaches are out there. Get one.

So, what about the clinical nurses out there? If we don't want to go into business, that doesn't mean that we have to do it all on our own. Even though we try, and yes- I have too, we don't have to be Super-Nurse catering to everyone's wants and needs.

At work, we can delegate tasks out to our support staff. We can talk to our peers when we are faced with a difficult case. Our managers, clinical specialists and educators are there to listen to what's going on with our lives. People are out there; we just need to reach out and ask.

We can even take this a step further and bring the tool to our home lives. If we are a busy nurse who works 50+ hours a week, maybe we need some help around the house. If we have a family, can we ask them to do a chore or two? Is there someone who can start dinner if we are going to be working late? Have you ever thought about actually paying someone for help? I know that housecleaning is not my strong suit and so I can choose to pay someone to come in and help. Gives them business too, right?

There is nothing demeaning or shameful about asking for help from another person. Think about you, as a nurse. You like to help people, right? How about letting some of those other people exercise their joy of helping others and allow them to help you from time-to-time?

Ask for and receive support. Even when you are not 100% clear of the question or need, just having the mindset that having support can help you is an asset to your forward progress. You don't have to go it alone.

Self-Reflection Exercises

Let's take some time here to delve into your comfort with asking for help. If you find it difficult or tend not to do it, why is that? Take a moment or two to write down some reflections and just think about the challenges you have with asking for support.

If you struggle with asking for support, can you shift that? Do you want to? What benefit do you see that may come from actually asking for help? Write those down.

Practice being honest with yourself and others. If someone comes up to you at work and asks you if you need help, take an assessment and answer with integrity. Let another person help you once this week and see how it feels.

Chapter 12
It's OK to Be You

Thank you for posting your question on doing the things that everyone else is doing.

My calendar (which I was so proud of and was so pretty with its color coding) was the 'everyone else' calendar. I am so thankful that you asked that and then that Alicia I could discuss further to make my OWN calendar ROCK!

Oh yes, and I'll have to redo it so that I can creatively and artistically color code and make it fun again!

Debbie's response: "Awesome job, Elizabeth. That is cool and courageous! I feel the same conversation coming up too.

I think my original goals were made (by me) to push myself in order to pace with others. The closer I am getting to my goal date, the more I realize that it's not going to happen. If I do force it, I will be totally out of the integrity with the work-life balance theme that I am trying to convey to my market that the work will be only adequate, which might lead to feelings of not being good enough...etc....

So, the key for me at least, is creating doable goals that will challenge me and yet will allow me to create and be in control.... like a good CEO. Basically, what I say to you is...."You go girlfriend!" Woo Hoo!!!"

Every year our coaching group goes through a strategic planning day. I actually enjoy planning things out so much, that one year, I took a huge cardboard rectangle and made an entire year calendar on it (just the months, I'm not that crazy). So, I had planned out everything I was going to do and had all of these goals, dates and marketing schemes laid out. Then, I did something completely unlike me. I totally trashed it.

My entire year was thrown out. Why? How come I wasted all of that good work that I had done? I realized that what I had put on that cardboard box was really not my calendar. It was what I had watched other coaches do; it was what other people in my coaching group had planned. It wasn't me.

Something I hear a lot as a nurse entrepreneur is this thing called the 'bright shiny object syndrome'. What this means is that you go after every 'new thing' out there. You want to take every class; you sign up for every training; you attend every event. Well, what happens when we act like this? We lose our sense of self.

This chapter's tip is simple. (What's that? What's simple isn't always easy; I know.) This chapter I encourage you to be yourself. Being your authentic self is the number one way to success. In business and in life.

It's hard to keep up with everyone. It's demoralizing to compare ourselves to the success of others. We put ourselves down when we try to do and become things that we are not. It's exhausting.

Yes the saying, 'fake it until you make it' surely does apply in business. If you are just starting out and you haven't worked with a single client yet, you may need to put on some confidence in order to get that first sale. But, do it *your* way.

Show up as yourself. People can tell when we are being an untrue representation of ourselves. Since everything is energy (including thoughts, feelings, words and actions) people pick up on that 'vibe' if you are being inauthentic.

This can ring true for those of us reading who are not yet, nor don't desire to be, entrepreneurs. At your workplace, are you being you? I see this a lot in nursing and I wrote about it a bit in Chapter Three of '*Nursing from Within*'.

Sometimes, our greatest asset can also be our biggest downfall. Millions of people around the world are nurses. Representing each specialty in healthcare and showing up in every level of care, nurses are everywhere. While this large group can be an asset as it provides us with colleagues, networks and camaraderie; this group notion can trip us up if we aren't careful.

We start to think like a nurse. Talk like a nurse. Act like a nurse. (Well, duh. We're nurses.) What I am warning you of is losing your sense of self in the profession. Just because your coworker went back to school does not mean you have to. Sure, your colleague got certified in that specialty, but do you really want to?

Make decisions based on your desires and dreams. Do what you want in nursing because it serves you. Follow your heart in your career. The greatest way to be the best nurse that you can be is to be yourself.

Again, sounds simple. Yet is it easy? Add on the fact that many of us have our family members and friends. Many nurses have children or they take care of adult parents. Many nurses are active in their faith, communities and government. Nurses can be siblings, children and friends. When we wear all of these 'hats' sometimes we lose who we are deep inside.

One final aspect I'd like to touch on in this chapter relates to the work that we do and how to engage in a career that never has to feel like 'work' again. Sure, some of you out there reading may be thinking to yourself *'Yeah right. We always have to 'work'. How else will we pay the bills?'* What I am referring to is something deeper. Something that taps into this concept of being your true you.

Many of the great entrepreneurs out there do what they do because they love it, not because they have to. Seriously, people have made great fortunes and probably never have to work another day in their lives. Yet they continue to do so. Why is that?

They have done the introspection and self work. They have gotten really quiet and listened. They have figured out what makes them 'tick', so to speak. They have done one thing that all of us would love to do: turned their passions into their jobs.

When you take time to pause and go inside you can find out what it is that you truly enjoy. You can uncover your unique traits, skills and talents. Then, you bring these into the work that you do- really apply them in your j-o-b. Whether it is as an employee of an organization or not; it doesn't matter. What is important here is that you are doing something of service that you really love to do.

Last year I wrote a blog post about a bus driver. Then, I wrote a follow up post about a waitress. Now, what do a bus driver and a waitress have to do with nursing? Absolutely nothing (unless the bus driver drove a bus at a hospital or something like that). Why did I write these posts?

Well, I experienced these two people in my day-to-day life. I rode a shuttle to-and-from my part-time job and I observed this man. He drove the same route day in and day out. Now to me, that seemed quite boring. Not to this guy! He was out front of our bus, waving us on in the afternoon. He would search the bus for dropped items and stand at the parking garage exit with things he found, checking each car to ensure the owner found their possessions. He greeted us with a smile, word of welcome and joke each day. I mean this guy *LOVED* his job.

Why was that? He didn't view it as a job! He found something he was good at, that he enjoyed and that used his unique talents and skills. His authentic personality was able to shine through. I bet work never felt like work for him and he enjoyed his career every single day of his life. (The same goes with my waitress example and you can always visit my blog at www.elizabethscala.com and search out 'Ode to the Waitress' to read more about that.)

Whether you are in business for yourself or not, it is imperative for your success that you show up as you. There are lots of 'bright shiny objects' out there that can tempt you into something different than what it is that you truly want. Who it is you want to be? Make sure that when you make decisions you make them for yourself from within.

Self-Reflection Exercises

What is it that you like about nursing? Why do you do it each day (in whatever role that you do)?

What would you like to learn next as a nurse? Not what other people are learning or telling you that you have to learn; what is the next thing you would like to know as a nurse in your career?

Where would you like your nursing career to go? Where do you want to see yourself next year, three years from now, or ten years from now? Instead of following someone else's path- start to follow your own.

Chapter 13
Tying it All Together in the Very Best Way

Well, here we are.

Phew. Nine practical tools that you can apply in your nursing career are behind us. Nine tips that you can use in business or within your role in your organization. I hope that you were able to apply each piece of advice to wherever you find yourself in your nursing practice.

My intention truly is to share with you the resources that have helped me not only build my business, but have assisted me with the growth as a human being. I often say, and actually have heard other entrepreneurs out there echo this as well, being in business for myself has been the hardest thing that I have ever had to do. *And,* it's been the most rewarding in terms of helping me thrive as a spiritual being.

My final tip to you is my personal number one value. We all have values in life, at least I hope we do. When I contemplate what's important to me, it may sound selfish, but it's true: my number one value is fun.

I want to have fun in every single thing that I do. I want to have fun with family and friends. Fun at work. Fun with fun. I want to have fun as I learn and grow and heal and change. Fun is important to me and allows me to feel free.

So, my last piece of advice is to have fun with your work. Quit taking yourself too seriously (we all do it; I am raising my hand here too). Laugh once in a while. Laugh at yourself. Play. Be a child again. I think the very best thing I have gained from my two nephews is that feeling of being childlike once more.

I am blessed with the opportunity to have them come and stay with me for a couple of days in the summertime. They ask me questions all day. They are constantly chattering to each other, themselves and to anyone who will listen. They laugh and play and act silly. Watching them experience the world is such a joy for me and having them stay with me that first summer that they did reminded me to experience the world as a child again.

If work is becoming too hard for you or if you are no longer enjoying yourself, take a break. Take some time off and replenish yourself. Here's another plug for all of the health and wellness coaches out there (and there are many nurses out there becoming coaches, too). Go ahead and find yourself a coach. A life coach, wellness coach, health coach or even personal coach. Whatever kind you need.

Take some time to enjoy being you, to have fun with your nursing career. Life is way too short. It will be over before you know it. Don't miss the world and all of its beautiful opportunity by being upset with how things are going. If you're unhappy make a change and then enjoy the choices that you make. Have fun being you and enjoy your own company.

Let's recap. Here are the ten entrepreneurial tactics that you can apply to more thoroughly enjoy and absolutely excel in your nursing career:

Be OK with where you are RIGHT NOW. Be patient on the path to forward progress, while recognizing the growth behind you. When you are OK with where you are at now, and able to celebrate everything about that, you exude that energy out into the world.

Have a plan. Even while you live in the present moment you can have a plan for the future. Create a clear vision for what you want and stick to that as you go forward with decisions.

Continue to trust when the going gets tough. Let go of the 'how' and any attachment to expectation or outcome. Remember, patience is key.

Be of service. Shift from how you may help yourself and your career to how you may help those that you serve (remember, WIFT).

Be consistent and persistent in your follow up. People are busy and require more than one avenue to get and keep their attention.

Fight the fear and become/be aware of your numbers. Knowing your numbers empowers you to do something about it and take action steps to move forward.

Celebrate success. The more we focus on the joy- the more we receive. In every single situation there is a win.

Ask for and receive support. Even when you are not 100% clear of the question or need, just having the mindset that having support can help makes it easier.

Be yourself. There are TONS of bright, shiny objects out there- and the #1 way to success is your way.

Have fun!

I'd like to share one more gift with you, if I may. I didn't know how to cram it all in so I decided to create a bonus chapter. I wanted you to have some concrete tips that you could use in your daily life to start to shift your mindset and perspective. These are things I do and have seen great success with… are you ready to join me? Before the book comes to a close- one more chapter of resources for you.

Let's go…

Part Three

Just for Today: A Step-by-Step Guide to Career Bliss

OK, if you've come this far you're serious about shifting your nursing career and if you're still with me, you really want to make some lasting changes. That's what this final section is all about.

I went back and forth on how to include the content in the following bonus chapter. Do I piece it in throughout the book? Do I leave it out for a future writing? How can I share a process with my readers that I know works and will definitely provide them with outcomes?

You may be thinking, '*Now that is a bold statement. She* knows *this works and it is going to* definitely *provide me with outcomes. Sign me up!*' You got it. How do I know this? The content in the bonus chapter is exactly what I did. It's what I continue to do. And guess what? The more I do it, as often or as close to on a daily basis as I can, the greater results I see.

Are you ready to learn how to enjoy career bliss now and forever? Let's do this. Here we go…

Bonus Chapter:
10 Simple Steps for Nursing Career Joy...
On a Daily Basis!

Want to know the question I get asked the most? (You may have asked me or been thinking to ask me yourself, actually.) Here it is: *"Elizabeth, how do you do what you do? How have you gotten where you are? How can I do what you're doing?"*

While I don't believe in cookie-cutter systems, I am going to share my ten step process with you here. My reason is twofold (and no, it's not to get you all to stop asking me). For one, in the introduction of this book, I promised you results. I said that if you put the materials in this book into action, actually implemented what you learned, you would receive results. That's what this ten step process can do for you. Second, I just love teaching content!

Really; I want you to have as much as you can to go forward with after reading this book. My goal here is for you to enjoy your nursing career. Whether you decide to become a nurse entrepreneur or not, I want you to love what you do and have fun being a nurse each and every day.

As I've said above and throughout this book, take what serves you and leave the rest. Just because these ten steps have worked for me, doesn't mean that each and every one is for you. I'll share here what has helped me shift my mindset in the very best of ways. You can decide if these items are for you. Ready? Let's get to it...

A Literal Glimpse into the Life

OK. I am literally going to walk you step-by-step through my morning and daily routine. I do this as close to daily as I can. When I am not on the road or away visiting family, if I am working in my home office, I do these steps. Some of them I can take with me as I travel. Yes, I really *can* do all of them away from my house as easy as I do them when I am home. But, just to be quite literal here- you're getting a glimpse into the life of Elizabeth Scala...

Step One: Out of Her Head!

During my studies at the Institute for Integrative Nutrition, I was introduced to a wonderful author and workshop leader. Julia Cameron wrote the book '*The Artist's Way*' and I highly recommend it.

I do what she suggests in her text. First thing in the morning (well, after I go to the bathroom and let my doggie do the same), I go to my journal. I write for three pages. When I say 'write', I mean write. No typing. No computers. No digital devices. I write for three pages- whatever comes to mind.

Maybe I write about my business; maybe about my dreams from the night before. Sometimes I write about a passage in another text I have alongside me. Or I just ramble on about nonsense because I cannot think of anything to write. It doesn't matter. The first step is to just get out of my own head and let whatever comes find itself on the paper.

Step Two: Enhance Awareness

This next step is critical to everything that has been previously written in this book. I've been saying it over and over again. Our thoughts, feelings, words and actions impact the outcomes we experience in our lives. I wrote a bit about my 'waking up' to meditation in my first book, *'Nursing from Within'*. It's a great story so I will share briefly about it here.

We had an all-day workshop at my hospital one year. I think it was on Tai Chi in healthcare. I went and was totally captivated by the speaker. Well, I contacted him after the fact and asked if he might train me some on holistic practices. I went to his office a few times. The final trip was a life lesson learned.

On my way to his office, my mind was racing. I was thinking about a class I had been teaching and how I feel the energy of people around me, and all sorts of things. Literally, I could not stop thinking. Well, I must have appeared that way when I showed up, because he actually put aside the lesson of the day and told me one thing.

"You need a meditation practice. Everything I teach you here will only be in vain if you can't get your mind to settle. Here's what I want you to do and you must do it on a daily basis."

He went on to teach me… I never went back to his office. And- my life has never been the same since…

The second step in my self-care routine involves mindful breath work. I literally sit on a block, with my hands in a certain Mudra, and I watch my breath. In the most basic terms, this is meditation.

Now you can find any type of meditation that works for you. Maybe it is the simple practice of watching the breath. Maybe you will enjoy chanting, humming or focusing on a single word. Maybe you will do a walking meditation. I don't care what it is…as long as you meditate.

There is no way you will be able to accomplish any of what we have discussed in the previous chapters of this book if you are distracted, consumed, overwhelmed or unfocused. I'm sorry. There's just no other way around it. It's absolutely imperative that you find a meditation practice that works for you-and stick to it.

Step Three: Get Clear

Now, this one may or may not be something you need to do on a daily basis. However, it is important that if you have not yet done so you, set aside the time to implement this step. Step three is about getting clear with what it is that you truly want out of life.

I have noticed that when I am not 100% clear; I don't get the results I want. As a nurse entrepreneur, I have to be on social media. Now we've talked about getting out there and that sort of thing in prior chapters, yet here's a perfect example that recently happened to me that will illustrate this for you.

I was working with a social media team for about six months. All in all, I was satisfied. I was happy with the price, yet not blown away with the work. I had this nagging feeling, this sneaky suspicion that this wasn't the right fit for me.

I shared my unsettling thoughts with my coach. She suggested a woman she had used in the past who she highly recommends. Well, I actually knew of this person because I had been watching her for a few years myself. I contacted her and we had a call; but something still didn't feel 100% accurate.

Well, as she always does, my coach had a brilliant idea. 'Elizabeth, why don't you write up what you're looking for and then send that intention out?' Funny thing was I had done that about a year or so prior; I just never did anything with it.

I actually pulled up the draft of the document I had created before and edited it to reflect where I was currently at. I put a header and footer on it and created a PDF. Then, I put it into a few nursing groups I was a part of and POOF! In minutes I had several responses. Good ones, too. I was thrilled.

Well, duh! What did I expect? When I was all over the place, I got all over results. When I slowed down and became clear; I got what I wanted!

It's amazing how quickly the universal laws deliver. The above example highlights that fact. It was literally within a matter of seconds that I started to receive responses on my post. Ask and ye shall receive, right?

So, this step is crucial for you as well and again, maybe you don't need to do this one every day. However, I do suggest that on a quarterly basis (at the very least), you check in with yourself and make sure you are clear on what you do want vs. what you don't want. The more clarity you can ask with, the quicker you will receive the results you desire.

Step Four: Visualize How You Feel

This next step is a really fun one. What I like to do is tack it onto the end of my mindful breath practice from step two. As I am sitting quietly on my block, I find that this is a good time to do my daily visualization.

Now, for those of you out there who are thinking to yourself, '*I can't visualize!*' - fear not. I have a hard time too. So I do the best I can. Even if I cannot 'see' a visual picture in my mind's eye (that space between your eye brows), I practice. My husband is actually *great* at visualizing and that irritates me a bit! But then again, he has to be for his job since he has to draw out what type of heating and air conditioning units are best for the spaces he puts them into.

Again, don't worry if you're not the best at seeing things inside of your head. What's important in this step is that you feel the benefits of your visualization. So how do you do this?

OK, to be quite literal, you build upon step number three. You hold in your mind's eye (or heart, or wherever you can) the visualization of what you want your life to be like. You call it up inside of your being. Then you picture what that desired life will actually feel like. It's as if you are experiencing the future, desired life in the current moment.

What will that feel like for you? How will you act? What will you be involved with; what will you be doing each day? Sit and visualize how the ideal life will feel for you.

Step Five: Connect with the Source

I love this next step. I learned this from a webinar and subsequent video training I went through with Kristen Howe. She suggested that we connect with our higher self on a daily basis and allow this light of spirit to fill our being. (Yikes, that all sounds very odd and new-agey, doesn't it?) To eliminate some of the 'woo' in this, let me share the practice I learned from her and do on a daily basis.

To do this exercise, Kristen taught us that it wouldn't take long and that it had to be done around a time we were quiet and still. Perfect, I thought to myself; I'll do this alongside my daily breath work. So that's what I've done.

OK, picture me sitting there on my block. I've done my meditation. Then I've spent some time visualizing and feeling (doesn't have to be long; five minutes in visualization is plenty for a day). Now, still sitting on the block, I open up myself to the divine.

I picture (well, for me 'picture' may not be the right word) the top of my head opening up. I allow a white light (feeling of the divine?) enter from above. This connects me to the universal sense of great support and abundance. I then move my attention (or that white light, if you are able to visualize it) down to my heart center, pausing a moment, before moving it out of my sits bones. That connected support (the white light, for those of you who can do this) travels down into Mother Earth, wrapping around the core, before coming back up to little old me sitting there on the block.

I am now enveloped with universal support from above, from within and from below. I feel the connection with divine source, my heart center and that of nature. It's a great way to sense that we are never alone and that love is all around us. It's a step that doesn't take very long to do, but is so beneficial to get into practice of feeling the loving guidance and support each day.

Step Six: Affirm with a Smile

OK. You can finally get off of the block. Phew! My tushie, right? But yes, you don't have to sit on the block any longer if you don't want to. It's time to open your eyes.

The next step involves a mirror. I also like to stand for this part. When I stand up, shoulders back and head high, I feel empowered. It's like being in the Mountain Pose from Yoga. And what do I do? I look into my own eyes, with a great big smile on my face, and I read my intentional affirmation statements.

Since this book isn't about creating affirmations and how to use them (you can find that in the supplemental workbook), I'll just share with you the process of what I am doing and how. I am looking into the mirror so that I can see into my 'self'. I am smiling so that I feel the benefit of the practice. I am speaking my intentional statements with affirmation to align my conscious and unconscious thought. This is a really effective step in my self-care system and, to be honest, I have seen probably some of the most beneficial shifts from this practice.

Step Seven: Listen from Within

Now this step may seem a bit 'out there' (maybe some of you are thinking that they *all* are), but I need a concrete way to tap into my intuition. Being more of a scientific, logical and analytical type person I have a hard time (or dare I say, I've had (as in the past) a hard time) hearing my intuitive self.

One of my spiritual teachers introduced me to card decks. Now there are tons of these all over and so what I suggest is find what works for you. What did I do? I literally went to Google (when I was at Cape May, NJ) and typed in 'crystal store'. That brought up a shop that had all sorts of self-help books, new age trinkets, inspirational CDs and card decks. When I went there, I meandered around the store for quite some time, just reading things and listening to what 'spoke' to me.

I purchased a few simpler decks (believe me, they can get quite intense) and now, during my morning practice (or at times when I just need some intuitive guidance), I simply ask myself. '*What energy shall I focus on today? What lesson do you have for me now?*' I pull a card and then read the passage that accompanies it (usually the basic decks have books that teach you how to read the cards). That's that. I go about my day and allow some guidance to lead me from within.

Step Eight: Bring the Steps to Life

This next step isn't really during any specific time of day, but rather is with me all day long. As I've been talking about throughout this book, the way to enjoy our nursing careers is through constant awareness and observation. It's about being accountable in one's life and realizing that we are conscious co-creators with a higher power.

So, step eight is watching my language and thought patterns throughout my entire day, as best I can. It's about looking at experiences and approaching them with a growth mindset. It's me learning from every experience, interaction and situation that arises. It's actually living the lifestyle I've been writing about in all of the pages that precede this one.

There's no magical wand that allows me to put this step into practice. It's a culmination of all of the above. It's continuing to do my daily practice in the peace and quiet- so that I can ultimately live it as consistently as I can in the real life experiences.

Step Nine: Tune into the Energy

As with the previous step, this one is about walking our talk. When we are mindful of universal laws and how they show up in our lives, we can tune into the vibrations of life. From the greater sense of higher self to Mother Nature herself, there are lessons to be learned all around us. We move ourselves forward deliberately whether it is through active action or passive inaction. We go with the flow of life.

Step Ten: Reflect and Renew

As of this writing, I now do this step all day long. I notice I do it while I walk my dog; I am aware of it as I drive in my car. I practice this out in public and alone during quiet reflection.

Step ten is about allowing for appreciation and creating a daily gratitude practice. For me, this started out at night. I used to keep a journal by my bedside (well, I still do- but as I just said, I tend to do this all day long now). Each night, before going to sleep, I write down three things I am grateful for that day. What's great about this practice is that there are many fun twists you can add to it.

I've learned from Lissa Rankin and Rachel Naomi Remen, in a tele-class I took with them, about a practice of reflection. They suggested we look for three things each day that inspired us, touched our hearts and made us feel awestruck. Another spiritual teacher shared with me that on top of the gratitude practice, we could look for something new to be thankful for each day. I've added my own little twist in terms of not only expressing thanks, but attaching to it how each gratitude actually makes me feel.

This step allows for some creative play. Find what works for you and get into the habit of practice. The most important thing about appreciation and gratitude is that you do it each day. This is a beautiful gift that helps you to rejuvenate and renew yourself on a daily basis.

The Time Has Come

In the words of Green Day, "*You don't have to go home, but you can't stay here.*" Our time together has come to a close.

I avoid using the word 'end' since (and another great line from that same song, 'Closing Time', boy those guys were on fire with that one) "*Every new beginning comes from some other beginning's end.*" We can move forward from our time here in this book to bigger and even better things.

My hope is that you take what you learned and implement something into your daily life. My goal is that your nursing career becomes and is the job of your dreams. I truly want you to feel like you never have to 'work' another day in your life.

Since we are at the end of our text, I wish you the best and you know I will never leave you hanging, so please be sure to check out the Appendix, About the Author and Special Invitation sections in this book. I'd love for you to keep me up-to-date on your progress in the *Your Next Shift* Facebook Group (Facebook.com/groups/YourNextShift) and even join me at a live event. Until we meet again... enjoy the day!

APPENDIX

Recommended Resources from Coaches, Teachers, Guides, Mentors and Colleagues:

B Is For Balance, Second Edition: 12 Steps Towards a More Balanced Life At Home and At Work by Sharon M. Weinstein

Confident Voices: The Nurses' Guide to Improving Communication & Creating Positive Workplaces by Beth Boynton

Feel the Fear . . . and Do It Anyway by Susan Jeffers

How Rich People Think by Steve Siebold

Law of Attraction Key: 5 Steps to Make the Law of Attraction Work for You by Kristen Howe

Mind Over Medicine: Scientific Proof That You Can Heal Yourself by Lissa Rankin

My Grandfather's Blessings: Stories of Strength, Refuge, and Belonging by Rachel Naomi Remen

New Nurse?: How to Get, Keep and LOVE Your First Nursing Job! by Caroline Porter Thomas

Nurses, Jobs and Money -- A Guide to Advancing Your Nursing Career and Salary by Carmen Kosicek RN MSN

The Artist's Way: A Spiritual Path to Higher Creativity by Julia Cameron

The Attractor Factor: 5 Easy Steps for Creating Wealth (or Anything Else) From the Inside Out by Joe Vitale

The LinkedIn Code: Unlock the largest online business social network to get leads, prospects & clients for B2B, professional services and sales & marketing pros by Melonie Dodaro

The Millions Within: How to Manifest Exactly What You Want and Have an EPIC Life! by David Neagle

The Nerdy Nurse's Guide to Technology by Brittney Wilson

The Path: Creating Your Mission Statement for Work and for Life by Laurie Beth Jones

The Power of Patience: How this Old-Fashioned Virtue Can Improve Your Life by M.J. Ryan

The Secret of Deliberate Creation by Dr. Robert Anthony

The ULTIMATE Career Guide for Nurses: Practical Advice for Thriving at Every Stage of Your Career by Donna Cardillo

UNconventional Nurse: Going from Burnout to Bliss! by Michelle DeLizio Podlesni

Your Career in Nursing: Manage Your Future in the Changing World of Healthcare by Annette Vallano

48 Days to the Work You Love: Preparing for the New Normal by Dan Miller

ABOUT THE AUTHOR

Spiritual Practice Nurse Elizabeth Scala is on a mission to shift the profession of nursing from the inside out.

Nurses typically enter their careers with a desire to provide compassionate, heart-based care. Challenged by regulations, financial pressures and technological advancements, todays nurse struggles to balance the art with the science of nursing.

As a keynote speaker, bestselling author, workshop facilitator and conference host, Elizabeth inspires nursing teams to reconnect with the passionate and fulfilling joy that once called them to their roles.

In addition to this book, Elizabeth has written and published several others you may enjoy. These books include:

Nursing from Within: A Fresh Alternative to Putting Out Fires and Self-Care Workarounds

Reiki Practice: A Nurse's Rx for Self-Care

Bring Back the ART of Nursing: Reconnect to Your Nurse Within

Learning through Experience: A Resource Book of Expert Interviews

Back to the Basics: A Nurse's Pocket Guide to Self-Care

Elizabeth is also a certified coach and Reiki Master Teacher. She lives in Maryland with her supportive husband and playfully, silly pit bull. When Elizabeth's not speaking to or teaching other nurses you can find her enjoying nature, relaxing on the beach, doing Yoga or dancing to her favorite jam band, moe.

You can find out more about Elizabeth at **www.elizabethscala.com.**

UP CLOSE & PERSONAL

Transform Your Nursing Career from Adequate to AWESOME

My fellow nursing colleague,

I don't know about you but I've met so many nurses who feel trapped by a profession that may or may not have their best interests at heart. Consider today's healthcare environment. Does it allow you to practice nursing the way that you want to?

Or do you find yourself, shift after shift, barely able to survive?

I bet this isn't how you imagined your nursing career would be. If your job isn't fulfilling your desire to use your nursing skills in a meaningful way… if it doesn't allow you to provide the type of care you know is best for your patients… then maybe it's time for a change.

Even though you may love the profession are you falling 'out of love' with your career?

If you find yourself answering yes, then please accept this invitation to Elizabeth's Live Workshop!

Take what you received in the pages of '*Your Next Shift*' and put it into practice at Elizabeth's In-Person Event, the '*Your Next Shift Workshop*'.

Reconnect to the passion and joy (*The Reason*) you went into the nursing profession in the first place

Feel energized and in love with your nursing career on a daily basis

Grab Your Greatly Reduced Ticket

As a reader of the 'Your Next Shift' book, I'm opening up the doors to my live event to you at an incredibly discounted rate!

Visit http://elizabethscala.com/events/ for information on the Your Next Shift live workshop and contact me at support@elizabethscala.com to cash in on your deeply discounted ticket today.